D0304098

SYNDROME IDENTIFICATION
for
Audiology

AN ILLU...   ...GU...

SYNDROME IDENTIFICATION
for
Audiology

AN ILLUSTRATED POCKETGUIDE

Robert J. Shprintzen, Ph.D.

Professor and Director
Communication Disorder Unit
Center for the Diagnosis, Study and Treatment
of Velo-Cardio-Facial Syndrome
Center for Genetic Communication Disorders
Department of Otolaryngology and Communication Science
State University of New York Upstate Medical University
Syracuse, New York

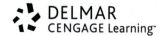

DELMAR
CENGAGE Learning

Australia • Brazil • Japan • Korea • Mexico • Singapore • Spain • United Kingdom • United States

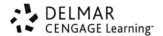

DELMAR
CENGAGE Learning

Syndrome Identification for Audiology: An Illustrated Pocketguide
Robert J. Shprintzen

Business Unit Director:
William Brottmiller

Acquisitions Editor:
Marie Linvill

Editorial Assistant:
Cara Jenkins

Executive Marketing
Manager: Dawn
Gerrain

Channel Manager:
Kathryn Bamberger

Executive Production
Editor: Barb Bullock

Production Editor:
Brad Bielawski

For product information and technology assistance,
contact us at **Cengage Learning Customer & Sales Support,**
1-800-354-9706

For permission to use material from this text or product, submit all
requests online at **cengage.com/permissions**
Further permissions questions can be emailed to
permissionrequest@cengage.com

Library of Congress Control Number: 00-049654

ISBN-13: 978-0-7693-0020-7

ISBN-10: 0-7693-0020-0

Delmar
5 Maxwell Drive
Clifton Park, NY 12065-2919
USA

Cengage Learning is a leading provider of customized learning solutions with office locations around the globe, including Singapore, the United Kingdom, Australia, Mexico, Brazil, and Japan. Locate your local office at: **international. cengage.com/region**

Cengage Learning products are represented in Canada by Nelson Education, Ltd.

For your lifelong learning solutions, visit **delmar.cengage.com**
Visit our corporate website at **www.cengage.com**

Printed in the United States of America
9 10 11 12 13   18 17 16 15 14

Contents

Preface

This, my second PocketGuide, has allowed me the opportunity to expand my continued interest in clinical genetics and dysmorphology by focusing my attention on disorders of hearing. As Director of a program in communication disorders within a department of otolaryngology at a major medical school and university hospital, I have had the opportunity to see hundreds of patients with congenital deafness or hearing loss. When I see newborns with identified hearing losses, I find myself wondering at what point the dramatic advances in molecular genetics will be translated into treatments that reach beyond the procedures currently employed. I have concluded that this is indeed an exciting time to be a part of the process that interfaces clinicians with molecular scientists. This volume is dedicated to that process and the hope that some of its readers will share my excitement and commitment to progress.

This PocketGuide is a compendium of multiple anomaly syndromes that have hearing loss as a major feature. Over 200 syndromes with deafness have been described, many of them rare or affecting only single families. In this book, I have tried to describe a solid core of syndromes with their total scope of communicative impairments. No list of multiple anomaly syndromes can be completely exhaustive because the fields of genetics and dysmorphology continue to expand at a rapid rate. I hope the reader will use this volume as a launching point for a continued interest in the genetics, developmental biology, and epidemiology of hearing loss. As nonsyndromic genetic hearing loss is not discussed in these pages, the reader is urged to explore this interesting field through other sources, including other comprehensive works. Of particular note is *Hereditary Hearing Loss and Its Syndromes* by Robert J. Gorlin, Helga V. Toriello, and M. Michael Cohen, Jr. The reader should also become acquainted with *Online Mendelian Inheritance in Man* (OMIM) which is a comprehensive web site describing all known genetic disorders in humans (http://www3.ncbi.nlm.nih.gov/Omim/). OMIM is free for anyone with internet access. I hope this volume will serve as an impetus for further study by audiologists and other scientists in this exciting age of discoveries in the fields of molecular and clinical genetics.

Each entry in this PocketGuide is structured to provide a brief description of the types of hearing loss and other communicative impairments that occur in association with the syndrome. These descriptions are largely based on the author's personal observations and clinical experience together with the known phenotypic spectrum of the syndrome. Extensive descriptions of hearing loss and communicative impairments do not exist for most syndromes and it is hoped that this volume will ignite the interest of clinicians to contribute to the process of syndrome delineation. Also listed in each entry is the etiology of the disorder as currently understood, and a comprehensive list of the anomalies associated with the syndrome. It is possible that some of the terms used to describe anomalies associated with the entries are unfamiliar to the reader. It is suggested that readers should utilize this PocketGuide as a road map to the world of multiple anomaly syndromes and that they continue to refer to other sources for additional information. New to this Pocket Guide is an entry for each syndrome, *Quick Clues.* Audiologists are typically in close contact with their patients, fitting headphones or ear inserts. Therefore, they have ample opportunity to notice obvious structural and behavioral abnormalities. Key diagnostic and easily noticed symptoms are listed under *Quick Clues.*

One caveat is offered regarding the etiologies listed. The study of genetically based syndromes is progressing at an unprecedented rate. The Human Genome Project has spurred an incredibly vigorous response to the study of human genetics and it is likely that a substantial amount of new information will be developed after the publication of this text. Every effort has been made to keep this information as current as possible, but new genes and the location and action of known genes are being discovered on a daily basis. Again, readers are urged to pursue their interest in genetics by referring to the Internet, OMIM, and professional publications.

Acknowledgments

The study of multiple anomaly syndromes is assumed by some to be a type of cataloguing of the strange and unusual. "Syndromologists" and dysmorphologists are often regarded as the "butterfly collectors" of genetics; people who keep collections of photos and case histories for the sake of learing more about abnormal patterns of development. I prefer to think of the process as more of a "Sherlock Holmesian" effort . . . the process of solving mysteries. In the end, the product of solving the mystery is making a diagnosis and understanding the implication of that diagnosis so better patient care can be rendered. Good detectives require the input of many experts in the process of gathering evidence. I would like to acknowledge a superb staff of audiologists and the otolaryngologists at Upstate Medical University in Syracuse who provide the continuing stream of detailed information necessary for being precise in the approach to diagnosis. They include audiologists Debbie Lightfoot, Andy Giraud, and Kathy Muldoon, and otolaryngologists Precha Emko, William (Bill) Harmand, Anthony (Tony) Mortelliti, Sherard A. (Scott) Tatum III, Charles I. (Sam) Woods, and my Chairman, Robert M. Kellman. Many thanks to these valued colleagues, clinicians, and scientists.

How to Use This Guide

The syndromes listed in this guide represent a group of disorders that will be encountered by audiologists because they result in disorders of hearing. The symptoms listed for each entry, although comprehensive, may not necessarily be entirely complete, simply because the continued study of rare disorders results in new discoveries over time. Furthermore, if a symptom is listed, this does not mean that an individual case will definitely express this problem. Each entry lists *possible* anomalies associated with the syndrome, and in some cases *probable* findings, but none are obligatory. However, the listing may present readers with problems that they may wish to check if they were not previously suspected. For example, some disorders listed in this PocketGuide have late-onset or progressive disorders that may not be suspected when individual cases are seen at a very young age.

The entries are listed in alphabetical order according to the nosology preferred by the author. The reader should be aware that many syndromes have more than one label, and the clinician may be more familiar with the other appellation. For example, Down syndrome may also be labeled as trisomy 21. Velo-cardio-facial has been called DiGeorge syndrome, CATCH 22, and conotruncal anomalies face syndrome. Because of these differences in the naming of various syndromes, alternative labels are also provided.

The natural history of each entry is also described. This refers to the expected course of the disorder over time. Clinicians should be aware that multiple anomaly disorders are rarely static in their presentation. Therefore, an individual clinician's experience with a specific disorder may be limited by the age of the case he or she has encountered. The presentation of Cockayne syndrome is a good example. Infants and toddlers with Cockayne syndrome are essentially normal, but early childhood brings the development of neurological, hearing, and visual deterioration. The clinician may wish to use these descriptions as a way of anticipating problems that may not have arisen as yet and to guide treatment to meet the expectations of the prognosis.

Abruzzo-Erickson Syndrome

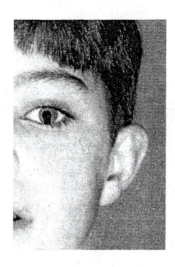

Abruzzo-Erickson syndrome: Iris coloboma is one of the major anomalies associated with this syndrome.

Also Known As:

This rare syndrome of hearing impairment (primarily sensorineural) also features craniofacial anomalies including cleft palate. The communicative phenotype can be confusing because the effects of the hearing impairment are superimposed on the resonance disorders that may accompany cleft palate. The presence of an ocular coloboma (cleft of the iris) may lead clinicians to suspect that patients with Abruzzo-Erickson syndrome have **CHARGE association.**

Major System(s) Affected: Craniofacial; growth; ocular; genital; musculoskeletal.

Etiology: X-linked recessive inheritance. The gene has not yet been identified or mapped.

Quick Clues: Coloboma of the iris is a relatively rare anomaly. The association of coloboma with hearing loss is found in both Abruzzo-Erickson syndrome and **CHARGE association,** but the auricular anomalies in Abruzzo-Erickson syndrome are different from those seen in

CHARGE with the ears being large and soft. The absence of heart anomalies is also a strong clue that the presence of the coloboma does not indicate **CHARGE association.** The presence of radial synostosis also differentiates Abruzzo-Erickson syndrome from **CHARGE association.**

Hearing Disorders: Hearing loss is typically mixed with a major sensorineural component. In some cases, the loss is purely sensorineural. The sensorineural component is potentially progressive and may become severe in adult years. In childhood, a 20–30 dB loss is more typical.

Speech Disorders: Speech may be affected by the hearing loss associated with Abruzzo-Erickson syndrome, and articulation may also be impaired from the effects of velopharyngeal insufficiency secondary to cleft palate.

Feeding Disorders: Other than the early effect of cleft palate, feeding is unaffected.

Voice Disorders: None.

Resonance Disorders: Resonance may be affected by velopharyngeal insufficiency secondary to cleft palate and may be exacerbated by hearing loss if the sensorineural component is severe.

Language Disorders: Expressive language is only affected if the sensorineural component of the hearing loss is severe.

Other Clinical Features:

> **Craniofacial:** cleft palate; large, soft auricles;
>
> **Growth:** short stature;
>
> **Ocular:** ocular coloboma;
>
> **Genital:** hypospadias;
>
> **Musculoskeletal:** radial synostosis.

Natural History: The anomalies in Abruzzo-Erikson syndrome are essentially static except for the hearing loss. The sensorineural component of the hearing loss may be progressive in some patients.

Treatment Prognosis: Intellect is normal and the general prognosis for normal speech and language is good depending on the severity of the sensorineural component of the hearing loss.

Differential Diagnosis: At the time the syndrome was delineated, there was speculation that Abruzzo-Erickson syndrome actually represented **CHARGE associ-** **ation.** However, there is no doubt that this condition is distinct from **CHARGE.**

Achondroplasia

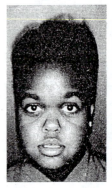 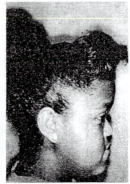 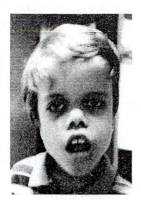

Achondroplasia: Note the midface deficiency and depressed nasal root. In the case shown at far right, note the chronic open-mouth posture indicative of upper airway obstruction.

Also Known As:

Achondroplasia is probably the most easily recognized genetic syndrome of short stature, especially short stature associated with disproportionately short limbs. The majority of cases are new mutations, but once the mutation has occurred, it is inherited as an autosomal dominant syndrome. Because there are many marriages between people of short stature, there have been homozygous cases (i.e., babies who have inherited two copies of the mutant gene, one from each parent). Homozygotes do not sur-

vive. Achondroplasia is a fairly common genetic disorder with a population prevalence of approximately 1:16,000 to 1:30,000. The exact frequency is somewhat difficult to calculate because other syndromes of short stature often resemble achondroplasia, and, in the past, the diagnosis was applied inappropriately because of the grouping of several different disorders.

Major System(s) Affected:
Growth; limbs; craniofacial.

Etiology: Autosomal dominant
inheritance caused by a mutation in

the *FGFR3* gene (fibroblast growth factor receptor 3) mapped to 4p16.3. The majority of cases represent new spontaneous mutations.

Quick Clues: The appearance of both the craniofacial complex and the limbs. The severe shortening of the midface with a very depressed nasal root makes the top of the cranium look disproportionately large even though cranial diameter often is increased. The limbs have limited extension at the elbows and the fingers are broad at the base and narrow at the tips so that the distal phalanges cannot be approximated when the fingers are held together.

Hearing Disorders: Conductive hearing impairment is commonly related to a number of factors, including chronic middle ear effusion, changes in temporal bone structure, and otosclerosis. Sensorineural hearing loss has been reported in a smaller percentage of cases, but is still relatively common. Skull shape can make the angulation of the ear canals abnormally steep with the location of the auricles set low.

Speech Disorders: Articulation impairment secondary to anterior skeletal open-bite is common in achondroplasia. In cases with neurologic impairment secondary to

hydrocephalus, there may be some neurologically based articulation impairment.

Feeding Disorders: Early airway compromise may contribute to failure-to-thrive. In later life, obesity is common.

Voice Disorders: Hoarseness is common in achondroplasia, and may be related to ossification of the laryngeal cartilages. Laryngeal position is also abnormal because of skull base anomalies.

Resonance Disorders: Hyponasality is very common in achondroplasia related to chronic nasopharyngeal obstruction. Abnormal oral resonance may also occur secondary to tonsillar obstruction of the oropharynx. The tonsils may be of normal size, but the entire pharyngeal airway is abnormally configured in achondroplasia so that the tonsils are often abnormally positioned.

Language Disorders: Language development is usually normal unless there are secondary neurologic complications from hydrocephalus.

Other Clinical Features:

> **Growth:** severe short stature (mean adult height is ap-

proximately 50 to 52 inches); osteochondrodysplasia; short limbs and digits (rhizomelic shortening); large head circumference; severe lordosis of the spine;

Limbs: restricted flexion of the elbows and hips;

Craniofacial: broad, prominent forehead; hydrocephalus; compression of the brain stem caused by abnormal stenosis of the foramen magnum; depressed nasal root; severe shortening of the anterior cranial base; cranial base kyphosis; strabismus.

Natural History: Although the manifestations of achondroplasia are obvious at birth, growth deficiency becomes more pronounced with age and the body more disproportionate to the limbs. Progressive stenosis of the foramen magnum can cause compression of the brain stem and spinal cord. Obstructive sleep apnea may become evident in late childhood or early adolescence, even if upper airway obstruction has not been noted in infancy. Obesity, which is common, may exacerbate the obstructive sleep apnea.

Treatment Prognosis: The articulation impairment seen in achondroplasia is related to the skeletal anomalies of the cranial base, which results in abnormal position and angulation of the lower jaw in relation to a short and hypoplastic maxilla. The articulation errors are obligatory in nature and will not typically resolve with speech therapy alone. However, orthognathic or craniofacial surgery may correct the anomaly, and the articulation impairment may resolve spontaneously, or with some speech therapy after surgery. The neurologic manifestations of the syndrome also require surgical intervention.

Differential Diagnosis: There are many syndromes with disproportionate shortening of the limbs in relation to a more normal trunk size, including pseudoachondroplasia, achondrogenesis, diastrophic dysplasia, hypochondroplasia, and Ellis-van Creveld syndrome.

Acrocallosal Syndrome

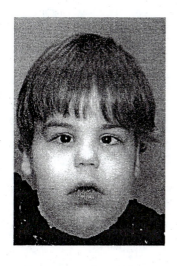

Acrocallosal syndrome: Note depressed nasal root and strabismus.

Also Known As: Schinzel syndrome, ACLS.

Acrocallosal syndrome was first delineated by Swiss geneticist Albert Schinzel in 1979. Although a rare disorder, it has sufficient overlap with other multiple anomaly disorders that some cases may have been misdiagnosed. Severe cognitive impairment is the rule and many patients do not develop intelligible speech.

Major System(s) Affected: Central nervous system; limbs and digits; craniofacial; cardiac; genitals; growth; abdominal.

Etiology: Autosomal recessive inheritance, mapped to the short arm of chromosome 12.

Quick Clues: The association of polydactyly with severe mental retardation and short stature is found in a small number of disorders, including acrocallosal syndrome. The presence of polydactyly in such cases with sensorineural hearing loss should alert the clinician to the possibility of acrocallosal syndrome in the differential diagnostic process.

Hearing Disorders: Sensorineural hearing loss has been reported in a few cases.

Speech Disorders: Many individuals with acrocallosal syndrome do not develop intelligible speech because of severe cognitive impairment. Cleft lip and palate occurs in over 10% of cases, which may further impair speech intelligibility.

Feeding Disorders: Severe hypotonia in infancy may result in a poor suck, but no other problems have been reported.

Voice Disorders: No voice disorders have been observed or reported.

Resonance Disorders: Hypernasal resonance may be present in cases with clefts.

Language Disorders: Severe language impairment is a constant feature of the syndrome.

Other Clinical Features:

Central nervous system: absence of the corpus callosum; arachnoid cysts; severe mental retardation; seizures; hypotonia; cortical atrophy;

Limbs and digits: preaxial polydactyly (duplication of the hallux); postaxial polydactyly; soft tissue syndactyly of two or more toes;

Craniofacial: macrocephaly; frontal bossing; prominent occiput; large anterior fontanel; hypertelorism; cleft lip and palate; depressed nasal root; strabismus; posteriorly rotated ears;

Cardiac: congenital heart anomalies;

Genitals: hypospadias; cryptorchidism;

Growth: short stature;

Abdominal: inguinal hernias; umbilical hernia.

Natural History: Growth deficiency is of postnatal onset and proportional. Neurologic and cognitive deficiency is apparent from infancy and initially presents as hypotonia. Seizures may also be apparent from infancy.

Treatment Prognosis: Depending on the severity of the central nervous system malformation, the prognosis for cognitive and language development is poor, as is the prognosis for normal speech development.

Differential Diagnosis: Hypertelorism, genital abnormalities, and clefting are common features of **Optiz syndrome,** which does not have as severe a developmental impairment. Clefting and polydactyly occur in several of the oral-facial-digital syndromes, some of which also have severe developmental impairment as a feature. Craniofacial anomalies, developmental impairment and polydactyly are also found in Carpenter syndrome.

Albers-Schönberg Syndrome

Also Known As: Osteopetrosis, autosomal recessive type; marble bones, autosomal recessive type; Albers-Schönberg disease.

There are two forms of Albers-Schönberg syndrome. The first, more familiar, form is a recessively inherited, severe, progressive bony overgrowth syndrome that has a poor long-term prognosis. The second form is a milder dominantly inherited form. Speech and hearing disorders progress as secondary manifestations of bony growth that impinges on the cranial nerves and mastoid bone.

Major System(s) Affected: Skeletal; craniofacial; central nervous system; ocular; dental; hematologic.

Etiology: Autosomal recessive inheritance; the gene for the recessive form has been mapped to 11q12-q13. The dominant form has been mapped to 1p21.

Quick Clues: The association of increased head size with progressive visual impairment, particularly when accompanied by nystag-mus, should raise the suspicion of Albers-Schönberg syndrome.

Hearing Disorders: There is progressive mixed or sensorineural hearing loss related to auditory nerve compression and progressive osteopetrosis, which alters the ossicles and temporal bone.

Speech Disorders: There is progressive compression of multiple cranial nerves, including VII and VIII, which can lead to paresis of facial animation and movement resulting in articulatory distortions and oral resonance abnormalities. Delayed dental eruption may cause articulatory distortion. Hearing loss may also be progressive and cause abnormalities of speech production. Osteomyelitis of the jaws may also cause restricted movement.

Feeding Disorders: If expressed early (congenitally), failure-to-thrive may occur related to airway obstruction or cranial nerve abnormalities.

Voice Disorders: Early voice production is normal. Hoarseness may develop in late childhood.

Resonance Disorders: Early resonance is normal, but hyponasality may develop in childhood or adolescence.

Language Disorders: A small percentage of individuals with Albers-Schönberg syndrome have cognitive impairment and may have language delay or disorder. However, the majority develop normal language before significant progression of the disease.

Other Clinical Features:

> **Skeletal:** osteosclerosis; osteomyelitis;
>
> **Craniofacial:** macrocephaly;
>
> **Central nervous system:** hydrocephalus;
>
> **Ocular:** progressive visual impairment from compression of the optic nerve; strabismus; nystagmus;
>
> **Dental:** delayed dental eruption; rampant dental caries;

Hematologic: severe anemia; thrombocytopenia; pancytopenia;

Other: hepatosplenomegaly; early death (usually in second or third decade of life).

Natural History: The bony changes and anemia are progressive, creating a worsening of all symptoms and early death.

Treatment Prognosis: Long-term prognosis is poor.

Differential Diagnosis: There are many progressive bone disorders, including the craniotubular disorders (**craniometaphyseal dysplasia, frontometaphyseal dysplasia, craniodiaphyseal dysplasia, van Buchem syndrome,** and sclerosteosis) that have similar progressive features and comparable deterioration and symptoms. The blood disorders will help to differentiate Albers-Schönberg syndrome.

Alström Syndrome

Also Known As: ALSS; pigmentary retinopathy, diabetes mellitus, obesity, and sensorineural hearing loss.

Alström syndrome is a rare disorder, and is another in the list of syndromes that have the association of pigmentary retinopathy and hearing loss (such as **Usher syndrome, Refsum syndrome,** and the Bardet-Biedl syndromes). Both the eye findings and hearing loss are progressive.

Major System(s) Affected:
Ocular; endocrine; integument; musculoskeletal.

Etiology: Autosomal recessive inheritance. The gene has been mapped to 2p13.

Quick Clues: The onset of nystagmus in early childhood with the association of obesity is easily noticed and consistent with the diagnosis of Alström syndrome.

Hearing Disorders: Progressive sensorineural hearing loss with onset in childhood has been observed in all cases. The hearing loss is cochlear in origin. The majority of cases have shown the hearing loss by school age. Vestibular function is normal.

Speech Disorders: Early speech development is normal and is only subsequently affected by the onset and progression of hearing loss.

Feeding Disorders: There are no feeding disorders in Alström syndrome.

Voice Disorders: Voice is normal.

Resonance Disorders: Resonance is normal.

Language Disorders: Language development is normal.

Other Clinical Features:

Ocular: initial night blindness; nystagmus; initial loss of peripheral vision; optic atrophy; eventual chorioretinal atrophy; cataracts; eventual blindness;

Endocrine: diabetes mellitus; obesity; growth hormone

deficiency; menstrual abnormalities in females;

Genitourinary: renal anomalies; small testes in males;

Integument: axillary acanthosis nigricans; premature alopecia in males; hair loss in females;

Musculoskeletal: scoliosis.

Natural History: The onset of the visual and hearing problems is in preschool years with relatively rapid decline of vision and hearing. Cognition is normal. Renal dysplasia may result in shortened life span.

Treatment Prognosis: The visual and hearing impairments have no known definitive treatment.

Differential Diagnosis: The features of Alström syndrome are similar to those of the subtypes of the Bardet-Biedl syndromes with the exception of cognitive function, which is normal in Alström syndrome. The Lawrence-Moon syndrome also has the association of obesity and visual degeneration, but infrequently shows significant hearing loss.

Antley-Bixler Syndrome

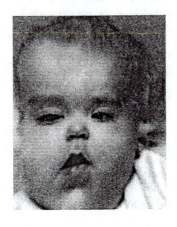

Antley-Bixler syndrome: Note the abnormal head shape, depressed nasal root, and ear abnormality.

Also Known As: ABS; trapezoid-ocephaly-synostosis syndrome; multisynostotic osteodysgenesis.

Antley-Bixler syndrome is a rare syndrome of craniosynostosis that has many extracranial anomalies, primarily involving the limbs and joints. The craniofacial anomalies are very severe and many infants with Antley-Bixler syndrome die in infancy from airway complications. External deformations of the auricles are common, including protuberant or cup-shaped ears. Microtia is not a feature of the syndrome.

Major System(s) Affected: Craniofacial; limbs; skeletal; genitourinary.

Etiology: Autosomal recessive inheritance. The gene has not yet been identified or mapped.

Quick Clues: The syndromes of craniosynostosis often have similar findings in the craniofacial complex, including midface deficiency, prominence of the forehead and calvarium, and distortion of the temporal bones. Antley-Bixler syndrome has distinctive limb anomalies not shared by other syndromes of craniosynostosis, such as femoral and ulnar bowing, rocker-bottom feet, and susceptibility to fractures.

Hearing Disorders: Conductive hearing loss is undoubtedly common in this syndrome, although

14

there have been no specific reports describing hearing in the syndrome. However, the degree of distortion of the temporal bones, reduced volume of the middle ear space, and Eustachian tube deformation is ubiquitous in the syndrome. Because many of the affected infants have died, the opportunity to observe the natural history of hearing loss has been limited.

Speech Disorders: Articulation is impaired by severe maxillary deficiency, Class III malocclusion, skeletal open-bite resulting in persistent tongue protrusion, severe restriction of oral cavity size, and nasal obstruction.

Feeding Disorders: Early feeding is impaired by respiratory compromise and nasal obstruction. As neonates with Antley-Bixler syndrome cannot breathe and eat simultaneously, their respiratory compromise must be dealt with prior to resolving their feeding problems.

Voice Disorders: None has been reported or observed.

Resonance Disorders: Hyponasality is common secondary to nasal obstruction, choanal atresia, or a small nasal capsule.

Language Disorders: Expressive language may be impaired, but there are patients with Antley-Bixler syndrome with normal cognition and intellectual development.

Other Clinical Features:

> **Craniofacial:** severe maxillary deficiency; depressed nasal root; frontal bossing; exorbitism; choanal stenosis or atresia;

> **Limb:** joint contractures of the elbows, knees, and digits; radiohumeral synostosis; femoral bowing; femoral fractures; ulnar bowing; rocker-bottom feet;

> **Skeletal:** rib anomalies; narrow iliac wings; hip dislocations;

> **Genitourinary:** female urinary tract anomalies and imperforate anus have been observed.

Natural History: As the various synostoses in Antley-Bixler syndrome are progressive, the craniofacial anomalies may become significantly more pronounced with age. Early death from airway obstruction occurs in a high percentage of patients with this syndrome, so aggressive treatment for airway obstruction, including tracheotomy, is indicated.

Treatment Prognosis: With early correction of airway obstruction, and eventual craniofacial surgery, there is the possibility that individuals with Antley-Bixler syndrome can develop normal cognition, speech, and language. However, many speech disorders are obligatory in nature and cannot be resolved with reconstructive surgery for craniofacial anomalies.

Differential Diagnosis: Several syndromes of craniosynostosis have unusual limb anomalies. Baller-Gerold syndrome has absence or hypoplasia of the radius and digital anomalies, but the craniofacial anomalies are not similar to those seen in Antley-Bixler syndrome. Craniosynostosis may accompany other syndromes with contractures, including arthrogryposis. Multiple synostosis syndrome may have similar limb anomalies in association with minor craniofacial anomalies. **Pfeiffer syndrome** has similar craniofacial anomalies with minor anomalies of the digits.

Apert Syndrome

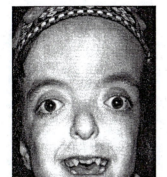
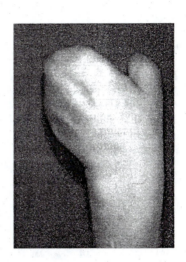

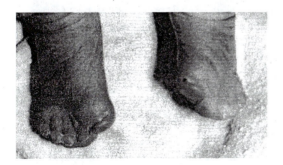

Apert syndrome: Note the orbital hypertelorism and anterior skeletal open-bite, and syndactyly of the hands and feet.

Also Known As: Acrocephalo-syndactyly.

Major System(s) Affected: Craniofacial; limb; central nervous system; growth.

Etiology: Single gene, autosomal dominantly inherited disorder caused by a mutation in the *FGFR2* gene (fibroblast growth factor receptor 2) located on the long arm of chromosome 10 at 10q26.

Quick Clues: The hand and foot anomalies in Apert syndrome are distinctive and essentially unique among syndromes of craniosynostosis. The characteristic "mitten hand" with the fusion of all or nearly all the digits should immediately point to Apert syndrome. The feet, although not as readily visible as the hands, are also distinctive with fusion of all or nearly all the toes and often a common nail across one or more of the toes. Because surgery is often done in early childhood to separate the digits, the clinician should look for scars on the hands and irregularities in the shape of the digits and the nails.

Hearing Disorders: Conductive hearing loss, usually mild to moderate, is common and may be re-lated to chronic middle ear disease, chronic fluid, ossicular anomalies, or any combination of the three. Progressive ossification of the ossi-cles and potential fusion may pre-sent as a progressive conductive hearing loss.

Speech Disorders: Articulation impairment related to malocclu-sion and open-bite with obligatory tongue placement errors results in anterior articulatory distortions. Because the maxilla is hypoplastic, the tongue often remains in the floor of the mouth with little or no articulatory placement in the max-illary arch.

Feeding Disorders: Upper air-way obstruction and possible cho-anal atresia may result in failure-to-thrive because infants with Apert syndrome will strive to maintain respiration even at the expense of feeding. In such cases, the airway obstruction must be relieved.

Voice Disorders: Hoarseness is occasionally present in childhood and adolescence, and may be re-lated to premature ossification of the thyroid, cricoid, or tracheal cartilages.

Resonance Disorders: Hy-ponasality is very common and

may be related to choanal atresia or stenosis, or to the small nasopharynx. In cases where cleft palate is found, mixed hyper/hyponasality may be present, but hyponasality is far more common.

Language Disorders:
Language delay is common and may develop with specific disorders related to cognitive deficiency. However, most children with Apert syndrome do develop adequate receptive and expressive language skills for communication. In the most severely affected cases, expressive language does not develop.

Other Clinical Features:

Craniofacial: synostosis of multiple cranial and facial sutures; maxillary hypoplasia; class III malocclusion; open-bite; cleft palate; choanal atresia or stenosis; small nasal cavity; orbital hypertelorism; low set posteriorly rotated ears; synostosis (fusion) of one or more ossicles; fixation of the footplate of the stapes; reduced size of middle ear space; chronic serous otitis; Eustachian tube dysfunction caused by abnormal angulation of the Eustachian tube orifice and reduced diameter of the tube because of abnormal bone growth of the surrounding craniofacial skeleton;

Limbs: syndactyly of fingers and toes; brachymelia (short forearms); acne vulgaris;

Central nervous system: mental retardation, macrencephaly, hydrocephalus, increased intracranial pressure;

Growth: occasional short stature.

Natural History:
Newborns with Apert syndrome have variable expression of the craniofacial findings, but fusion of all the digits on all limbs occurs in most cases. Choanal atresia or stenosis results in early airway obstruction and possible severe obstructive apnea, which may require emergency treatment, including possible tracheotomy. Craniofacial findings progress following birth and abnormal craniofacial growth becomes evident early in life, usually before two years of age. In some cases, craniofacial findings are severe at birth. Developmental delay is common, although some patients have normal cognition and development. In some cases, however, cognitive impairment is severe.

Class III malocclusion with developing open-bite is often evident by school age. Craniosynostosis continues after birth resulting in progressive distortion of the cranial bones and progressive midface hypoplasia. Learning disorders are usually evident early in life and mental retardation or learning disabilities often result in special class placement. The majority of children with Apert syndrome have some type of cognitive impairment. Life expectancy is normal.

Treatment Prognosis: Articulation disorders associated with Apert syndrome in childhood will be resistant to speech therapy because of the structural anomalies of the oral cavity. The errors are obligatory and will not be expected to resolve without surgical reconstruction of the craniofacial skeleton with craniofacial and/or orthognathic procedures. Language impairment will often respond to treatment, but progress may be limited by cognitive impairment. Hyponasality is also obligatory and can only be resolved with surgical management of the midface hypoplasia. Choanal stenosis or atresia are typically resistant to surgical resolution because of progressive skeletal dysplasia and because children with Apert syndrome are chronic mouth breathers. Lack of nasal respiration will prevent the nasal cavity from remaining patent, even after surgical repair. Hearing loss will also necessitate surgical resolution.

Differential Diagnosis: There are several other syndromes which have the association of craniosynostosis and limb anomalies, including **Saethre-Chotzen syndrome, Pfeiffer syndrome, Jackson-Weiss syndrome,** and Shprintzen-Goldberg syndrome. Though the craniofacial anomalies in these syndromes are similar to those seen in Apert syndrome, only children with Apert syndrome have the "mitten hand" resulting from the syndactyly of all the fingers or fusion of all the toes. **Crouzon syndrome** has similar craniofacial anomalies, but no syndactyly. Interestingly, **Jackson-Weiss** and **Crouzon syndrome** are caused by a different mutation in the same *FGFR2* gene as Apert syndrome.

Beckwith-Wiedemann Syndrome

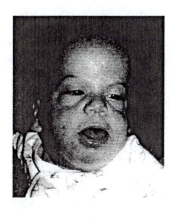

Beckwith-Wiedemann syndrome: Prognathism and macroglossia in an infant with Beckwith-Wiedemann syndrome.

Also Known As: Wiedemann-Beckwith syndrome; exomphalos-macroglossia-gigantism syndrome (EMG syndrome).

Beckwith-Wiedemann syndrome is a relatively common multiple anomaly syndrome, perhaps the most common overgrowth syndrome in humans, with a frequency of approximately 1:13,000 live births. Although hearing loss is not considered one of the prominent features of Beckwith-Wiedemann syndrome, it does occur frequently as a secondary finding to chronic middle ear effusion. Because essen-tially all children with Beckwith-Wiedemann syndrome have speech and language impairment (typically mild), the concurrence of hearing loss places these children at high risk for global communicative impairment. The syndrome is almost always detected initially in infancy because of abdominal abnormalities, metabolic disorders, or overgrowth coupled with hypotonia. It should be of particular interest to speech-language pathologists because of macroglossia and mandibular prognathism coupled with hypotonia, which causes a wide array of articulation disorders. Cleft palate, including a high prevalence of submucous cleft palate, may further complicate speech disorders.

Major System(s) Affected: Growth; craniofacial; gastrointestinal/abdominal; metabolic/endocrine; genital, motor development; central nervous system.

Etiology: Autosomal dominant inheritance. Several mechanisms for the disorder have been reported, including a contiguous gene duplication, uniparental disomy, and imprinting related to absence of a maternal copy of a gene. The locus for the syndrome has been isolated to 11p15.5. A gene called *IGF2* (insulin growth factor 2) has been implicated, but does not seem to explain the full range of anomalies in the syndrome.

Quick Clues: Overgrowth and hypotonia occur in a number of syndromes, including Sotos syndrome, Weaver syndrome, and the Golabi-Rosen syndrome. One of the hallmarks of Beckwith-Wiedemann syndrome is the history of omphalocele in many cases, and the presence of mandibular prognathism that is evident even in early infancy. Although Golabi-Rosen syndrome also shows mandibular prognath-

ism, omphalocele is not a clinical feature of that syndrome.

Hearing Disorders: Chronic middle ear effusion with conductive hearing loss is common, especially among patients with cleft palate. The problem is most common in infancy and early childhood.

Speech Disorders: Speech onset is often mildly delayed secondary to possible hypotonia and occasional mild developmental delay. Hypoglycemia is a common finding that can contribute to hypotonia and developmental delay. Articulation disorders are very commonly related to macroglossia and malocclusion. Patients with Beckwith-Wiedemann syndrome are typically prognathic and also have dental spacing abnormalities. The presence of a large tongue together with jaw and dental anomalies results in obligatory anterior articulation errors of distortion or compensatory placement errors. The tongue may articulate in the mandibular arch rather than the maxillary arch for lingua-alveolar sounds because of the macroglossia. Cleft palate or submucous cleft palate is a fairly common finding in Beckwith-Wiedemann syndrome and can complicate the articulation disorders. Because hypotonia is also common in the syndrome, children with Beckwith-Wiedemann syndrome who have cleft palate and velopharyngeal insufficiency are very likely to develop compensatory patterns, including glottal stop substitutions, pharyngeal fricatives, and pharyngeal stops. Many patients with Beckwith-Wiedemann syndrome also have hypertrophic tonsils and/or adenoids which may cause a chronic mouth-open, tongue forward posture, aggravating the macroglossia and hypotonia and resulting in fronting errors.

Feeding Disorders: Early feeding in the neonatal period is occasionally complicated by hypotonia and macroglossia. Airway obstruction is common, resulting in early failure-to-thrive.

Voice Disorders: Hoarseness of unknown etiology has been observed in some patients.

Resonance Disorders: Hypernasality is possible in individuals with cleft palate. If hypotonia is present, hypernasality is more likely to develop. Hyponasality may also occur secondary to adenoid hypertrophy, and mixed hyper/hyponasality may also occur in patients with hypertrophic tonsils and adenoids. Oral resonance may

also be impaired by hypertrophic tonsils.

Language Disorders: Language development is variable and depends on the presence or absence of cognitive impairment. Intellect is often normal, but mild impairment or borderline cognition is not uncommon.

Other Clinical Features:

>**Growth:** overgrowth; hemihypertrophy;

>**Craniofacial:** large mouth; mandibular prognathism; macroglossia; cleft palate;

>**Gastrointestinal/abdominal:** omphalocele; prune belly; umbilical hernia; enlarged liver;

>**Metabolic/endocrine:** neonatal hypoglycemia; anomalies of the renal medulla; adrenocortical cytomegaly;

>**Motor development:** hypotonia (may be secondary to hypoglycemia);

>**Central nervous system:** occasional cognitive impairment; seizures (not common); hydrocephalus (not common);

Genital: enlarged genitalia (male and female);

Other: development of neoplasias, including Wilms' tumor; adrenal carcinoma nephroblastoma, among others; cardiomyopathy; abnormal creases on the ear lobes and indentations on the back of the ear.

Natural History: The neonatal period is complicated by hypotonia, which may be secondary to hypoglycemia. The hypoglycemia resolves over time and there is significant catch-up of developmental milestones. The developmental, speech, and language phenotypes improve over time, but patients must be screened frequently for the development of neoplasias, particularly Wilms' tumor. The early overgrowth eventually plateaus, and after puberty, growth slows so that individuals with Beckwith-Wiedemann syndrome do not have adult gigantism.

Treatment Prognosis: The prognosis is excellent for normal speech and language.

Differential Diagnosis: Overgrowth is a feature of a number of syndromes which may also have hypotonia as an early feature, including Sotos syndrome. The presence of hypoglycemia and large birth size may resemble babies of diabetic mothers, a teratogenic effect. Hemihypertrophy and hemihyperplasia also exist as distinct syndromes. Omphalocele with facial anomalies and hypotonia has been reported in Shprintzen-Goldberg II syndrome.

Bloom Syndrome

Also Known As:

Bloom syndrome is a complex autosomal recessive genetic disorder of short stature and a high frequency of cancer that involves mutable chromosomal structure. Over 20 anomalies are associated with this syndrome, which is most common among Ashkenazi Jews of Eastern European origin. Nearly 1% of Israeli Ashkenazi Jews are gene carriers. The gene is far less common in other racial and ethnic subgroups.

Major System(s) Affected:
Growth; integument; craniofacial; immune; cardiopulmonary; metabolic/endocrine; reproductive; central nervous system.

Etiology:
Autosomal recessive inheritance. The gene has been mapped to 15q26.1.

Quick Clues:
The high-pitched voice in Bloom syndrome is distinctive, and when found in association with red patches on a blotchy skin surface and telangiectasias (small visible veins in the surface of the skin), Bloom syndrome should be suspected.

Hearing Disorders:
Conductive hearing loss secondary to chronic ear infections with middle ear effusions is common. The middle ear disease is often intractable with one infection following another, and may be in association with other respiratory illnesses, such as pneumonia, bronchitis, and croupe.

Speech Disorders:
Speech is typically normal, although in some cases there may be relatively late onset.

Feeding Disorders:
Neonatal feeding disorders have not been documented or observed. Adult feeding disorders may develop later if neoplasias occur in the digestive tract or if general vitality is reduced by chronic illness or cancer.

Voice Disorders:
Voice is high pitched and has been described as "squeaky."

Resonance Disorders:
Resonance disorders have not been reported or observed.

Language Disorders: Language development is typically normal, or only slightly delayed in some cases.

Other Clinical Features:

> **Growth:** short stature of prenatal onset; low birthweight;

> **Integument:** telangiectasias; erythema induced by exposure to sunlight; patches of both hyperpigmentation and hypopigmentation; café-au-lait spots;

> **Craniofacial:** micrognathia or retrognathia; malar hypoplasia; thin, triangular face; dolicocephaly; prominent nose;

> **Immune:** chronic upper and lower respiratory infections;

> **Cardiopulmonary:** pulmonary insufficiency; cardiomyopathy;

> **Metabolic/endocrine:** diabetes mellitus;

> **Reproductive:** sterility; testicular hypoplasia; cryptorchidism;

> **Central nervous system:** learning disabilities;

> **Other:** very high frequency of neoplasias, especially leukemia, lymphoma, and skin cancers.

Natural History: Following low birthweight, growth velocity remains steady, but height and weight remain low throughout life. Neoplasias typically develop in adolescence or early adult life. As a result of chronic infections, respiratory disorders, and the frequency of neoplasias, life expectancy is often dramatically shortened. With age, there is a high frequency of chromosome breakage and sister chromatid exchange of genetic material, which may lead to somatic mutations and the high frequency of neoplasias.

Treatment Prognosis: The administration of growth hormone has shown promise in increasing height. It is unclear if there is a positive effect on voice production, but it is likely that with increased stature and growth, vocal pitch may normalize.

Differential Diagnosis: There are a number of syndromes that show a high frequency of neoplasias in association with short stature, immune disorders, and skin lesions, including **Cockayne syn-**

drome and Rothmund-Thompson syndrome. Unlike Bloom syndrome, **Cockayne syndrome** is marked by severe cognitive impairment with rapid deterioration in adult life. Rothmund-Thompson syndrome has significant limb anomalies, (such as severely hypoplastic thumbs) and dental anomalies.

BOR *Syndrome*

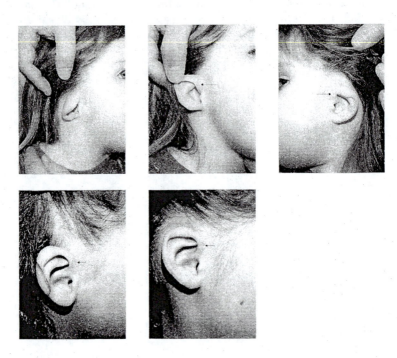

BOR syndrome: Note the preauricular fistulae (arrows) located anterior to the helix and above the tragus. Also note the lop ear anomaly.

Also Known As: Branchio-oto-renal syndrome; Melnick-Fraser syndrome.

As BOR is one of the more common syndromes of hearing loss, audiologists are almost certain to encounter such cases. Although BOR syndrome is relatively easy to recognize, it does show phenotypic overlap with a number of other common disorders and therefore is often misdiagnosed. Recognition of the syndrome is important because of the renal malformations that accompany the hearing loss and structural anomalies of the ear.

Major System(s) Affected: Auditory; craniofacial; renal; neck; pulmonary.

Etiology: Autosomal dominant inheritance. The gene has been mapped to the long arm of chromosome 8 at 8q13.3. The gene is labeled *EYA1*.

Quick Clues: The ear pits associated with BOR syndrome are distinctive in that they are typically located on the auricle just above the tragus, rather than in a preauricular position. This feature is found in only several other syndromes, including **Niikawa-Kuroki syndrome** (Kabuki syndrome).

Hearing Disorders: Hearing loss is probably the most common manifestation of BOR syndrome and may be either purely conductive, mixed, or sensorineural. Ear malformations are common in BOR, including anomalies of the external ear, external ear canal, middle ear, cochlea, and vestibular system. Anomalies of the cochlear nerve have also been identified. The most frequent type of hearing loss in BOR is mixed, because both conductive and sensorineural deficits are common. The degree of impairment ranges from mild to profound and is usually symmetric, but asymmetric cases have been seen. Hypoplasia of the apex of the cochlea has been documented in many cases, as has fixation of the footplate of the stapes.

Speech Disorders: Speech may be affected by mixed or sensorineural hearing loss. Cleft palate (often submucous) is also found in some cases and may lead to compensatory articulation disorders. Malocclusion, including anterior skeletal open-bite, lateral open-bite, or retrognathia is a fairly common finding, which may result in obligatory distortions or substitutions.

Feeding Disorders: Feeding disorders in infancy have not been considered a feature of BOR syndrome. There are no feeding impairments in childhood, adolescence, or adult life.

Voice Disorders: Voice is typically normal in BOR.

Resonance Disorders: Resonance may be abnormal based on the effects of sensorineural hearing loss and/or cleft palate. Cleft palate in BOR is most often submucous, and is therefore not detected in many cases.

Language Disorders: Language is typically normal in BOR, other than the effects of the more severe forms of hearing loss in some cases.

Other Clinical Features:

> **Auditory:** external ear malformations, typically small cup-shaped ears, or lop ears; ossicular anomalies, including stapes fixation; hypoplastic cochlear apex; vestibular anomalies; ear pits;

> **Craniofacial:** micrognathia; retrognathia; facial asymmetry; dental malocclusion; cleft palate;

> **Renal:** small or absent kidneys; cystic kidneys; anomalies of the renal collecting system;

> **Neck:** branchial clefts;

> **Pulmonary:** pulmonary hypoplasia.

Natural History: The hearing loss in BOR syndrome is typically static, but several cases of mildly progressive hearing loss have been observed. Cognition and motor development are normal. Early detection of kidney anomalies is important and treatment of the kidney problems associated with the malformations is possible.

Treatment Prognosis: The hearing loss in BOR syndrome is responsive to amplification. Air conduction hearing aids are applicable if the external ear anomalies permit proper fitting.

Differential Diagnosis: The presence of external ear anomalies associated with ear pits, hearing loss, and facial asymmetry is a common combination in BOR and is often mistaken for **oculo-auriculo-vertebral dysplasia (OAV,** or hemifacial microsomia). Because of this common diagnostic mistake, for many years children born with **OAV** (hemifacial microsomia) were often referred for examination of the kidneys and the collecting system (often with intravenous pyelograms). In true cases of **OAV,** positive renal findings would be rare, but in patients with BOR, kidney anomalies are common. Sensorineural hearing loss is far more common in BOR syndrome than in **OAV.** In addition, the ear pits in

BOR syndrome are located on the anterior edge of the auricle, but in OAV the pits or ear tags are preauricular. There are a number of rare syndromes of hearing loss with the association of ear pits and sensorineural hearing loss with other minor malformations, but the most common syndrome to be suspected should be BOR.

C Syndrome

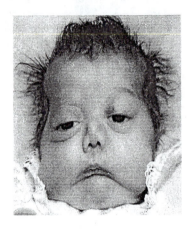

C syndrome: Note severe craniofacial anomalies, including trigonocephaly and proptosis.

Also Known As: Opitz trigonocephaly syndrome.

This is a rare autosomal recessive disorder with distinctive craniofacial anomalies, limb disorders, and mental retardation in those individuals who survive the neonatal period. Half or more of affected infants do not survive to childhood.

Major System(s) Affected: Craniofacial; limb; central nervous system; skeletal; cardiac; skin; genitals; ocular.

Etiology: Autosomal recessive inheritance. The gene has not been mapped or identified.

Quick Clues: Trigonocephaly is often seen as an isolated anomaly, but when the skull anomaly is severe and associated with marked developmental delay and polydactyly, the pattern becomes distinctively associated with C syndrome.

Hearing Disorders: As is true in most syndromes with craniosynostosis, conductive hearing impairment is likely to occur related to malformation of the cranium and temporal bones. Because of the high frequency of severe cognitive impairment and failure-to-thrive in C syndrome, it is likely that the specific nature of hearing loss has not been documented in many cases to date.

Speech Disorders: The cognitive impairment in C syndrome is severe and the development of speech is unlikely.

Feeding Disorders: Early failure-to-thrive is common and may be related to a number of factors, including severe hypotonia, airway obstruction, and heart anomalies.

Voice Disorders: Voice has not been assessed because of the lack of speech and language development.

Resonance Disorders: Resonance has not been assessed because of the lack of speech and language development.

Language Disorders: The cognitive impairment in C syndrome is severe and the development of expressive or receptive language is unlikely.

Other Clinical Features:

Craniofacial: trigonocephaly; metopic synostosis; microcephaly; upslanting eyes; depressed nasal root; epicanthal folds; micrognathia; posteriorly rotated ears; multiple oral frenula; soft tissue hypertrophy of the palatal shelves; broad maxillary alveolus; abnormal helical rims; occasional cleft palate;

Limb: polydactyly; syndactyly; short limbs; joint contractures; talipes equinovarus; joint dislocations;

Central nervous system: severe mental retardation; hypotonia; seizures;

Skeletal: short neck; hip dysplasia;

Cardiac: heart malformations;

Skin: lax skin;

Genitals: cryptorchidism; prominent clitoris in females;

Ocular: strabismus.

Natural History: At birth, head circumference and head shape are normal. Microcephaly and craniofacial growth anomalies progress after birth. Limb and joint abnormalities are evident from birth, and performance is impaired from birth. Approximately 50% of known cases have not survived infancy.

Treatment Prognosis: Poor.

Differential Diagnosis: A number of chromosomal rearrangement syndromes have trigonocephaly and microcephaly as common findings, including del(9p), del(11q), and dup(13q).

Cat Eye Syndrome

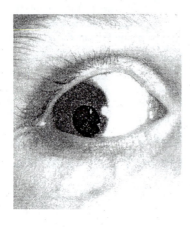

Cat eye syndrome: Iris coloboma in a patient.

Also Known As: CES; chromosome 22 partial tetrasomy; inv dup(22)(q11); Schmid-Fraccaro syndrome.

Cat eye syndrome is a disorder caused by a chromosomal rearrangement in the same region that causes **velo-cardio-facial syndrome (VCFS),** 22q11. Although the chromosome region is the same as in **VCFS,** the syndrome is distinctly different. The term "cat eye" was originally applied as a description of the iris coloboma that is a common feature in this syndrome.

Major System(s) Affected: Central nervous system; ocular; craniofacial; ears; cardiac; gastrointestinal; renal.

Etiology: Individuals with cat eye syndrome have extra chromosome material which is seen as a "marker" chromsome on karyotyping. The marker chromsome consists of the acrocentric short arm and a portion of the long arm of chromosome 22 to the q11 band. These markers have been demonstrated to be dicentric (two centromeres).

Quick Clues: The presence of coloboma of the iris immediately narrows down the differential diagnosis to a relatively small hand-

34

ful of disorders. The remaining features are quite similar to those found in **CHARGE association** and also overlap with **velo-cardio-facial syndrome.** Therefore, the presence of ocular colobomas in association with congenital heart disease should lead to the recommendation for laboratory analyses, including high resolution karyotype with focus on chromosome 22, and possibly fluorescent in situ hybridization (FISH) for a possible deletion of 22q11.2.

Hearing Disorders: Mild conductive hearing loss may occur secondary to minor auricular anomalies and narrowing of the external auditory canal. Chronic middle ear effusions often occur secondary to cleft palate.

Speech Disorders: Speech is affected by delayed motor development and incoordination that is variable, ranging from mild to severe. Cleft palate is also a common finding (at least 25% of cases) and may result in velopharyngeal insufficiency with compensatory articulation patterns.

Feeding Disorders: Early feeding may be impaired by hypotonia. Long term, there is no major feeding problem.

Voice Disorders: Voice disorders have not been reported.

Resonance Disorders: Hypernasality is common in cases with cleft palate.

Language Disorders: Language is typically delayed, usually mildly, although in cases with more severe cognitive impairment, a moderate to severe impairment is possible.

Other Clinical Features:

Central nervous system: cognitive impairment is common, ranging from borderline to moderate, although some cases with normal intellect have been documented;

Ocular: iris coloboma in at least 70%; microphthalmia;

Ears: small ears; protuberant ears; preauricular tags or pits;

Cardiac: tetralogy of Fallot; total anomalous pulmonary venous return;

Gastrointestinal: anal atresia or abnormal anal placement; malrotation of the gut; Meckel diverticulum;

Renal: hypoplastic or aplastic kidneys, unilateral or bilateral.

Natural History: The anomalies associated with cat eye syndrome are essentially static and late-onset findings have not been noted. Growth is typically normal, although some cases have mild postnatal growth deficiency.

Treatment Prognosis: The prognosis is dependent on the degree of cognitive impairment. Some infants with cat eye syndrome do not survive the neonatal period because of heart or renal anomalies, but the majority of patients survive and have a normal life span.

Differential Diagnosis: Ocular coloboma associated with ear anomalies, anal anomalies, and cognitive impairment is common in **CHARGE association** and may also be seen in **velo-cardio-facial syndrome.**

CHARGE Association

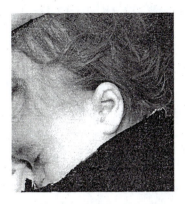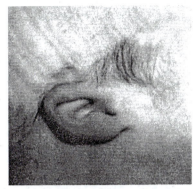

CHARGE association: Variation in ear anomalies associated with CHARGE.

Also Known As:

CHARGE is an acronym for Colo-boma, *H*eart anomalies, *A*tresia choanae, *R*etarded growth and development, *G*enital hypoplasia, and *E*ar anomalies. The term "association" refers to an etiologically nonspecific disorder that does not show clear evidence of being a sequence. Although a number of other syndromes have anomalies that fit the CHARGE acronym, there does seem to be a core of individuals with a consistent pattern that probably represents a distinct recurrent pattern syndrome.

Major System(s) Affected:
Central nervous system; craniofacial; growth; ocular; auditory; cardiac; skeletal; genital.

Etiology: The large majority of cases have been sporadic occurrences, but autosomal dominant inheritance has been observed. No genetic mutations, chromosome rearrangements, or teratogenic influences have been identified as causally related to CHARGE. A number of syndromes with known causation have clinical features consistent with CHARGE association, including **velo-cardio-facial syndrome**

and **Wolf-Hirschhorn syndrome.** A possible link to 14q22-q24.3 has been hypothesized.

Quick Clues: Coloboma of the iris is not a very common malformation, so its presence in association with hearing loss should raise a high level of suspicion regarding the possible diagnosis of CHARGE. An important visual clue is provided by the auricular anomalies, especially when asymmetric.

Hearing Disorders: Conductive, sensorineural, and mixed hearing loss have all been observed. In many cases, a trough-shaped mixed hearing loss is common, often affecting the speech frequencies most severely. Vestibular anomalies are also common.

Speech Disorders: Speech is almost always abnormal with multifactorial contribution to poor speech production. Articulation is impaired both by malocclusion and central nervous system impairment. Sensorineural hearing loss also adds to the mix of factors which results in unintelligible speech.

Feeding Disorders: Feeding is almost always impaired by multiple factors, including choanal atresia, hypotonia, developmental delay, and congenital heart anomalies. Some children have severe failure-to-thrive unless the cause(s) of the feeding difficulty is identified and resolved.

Voice Disorders: Hoarse or breathy voice is common and may be related to unilateral vocal cord paresis.

Resonance Disorders: Hyponasality is common, related to choanal atresia. In cases with cleft palate, there may be a mixed hyper-hyponasality, or a cul-de-sac resonance pattern related to the combination of velopharyngeal insufficiency with nasal obstruction. An abnormal oral resonance is also common, related to a short neck, small mouth, and hearing loss.

Language Disorders: Language impairment is very common and may often be severe. Verbal language may not be obtained by a significant percentage of patients because of the combination of cognitive impairment and hearing loss.

Other Clinical Features:

> **Central nervous system:** cognitive impairment; brain malformations;

Craniofacial: facial paresis; facial asymmetry; microcephaly; low-set posteriorly rotated ears; protuberant ears; prominent nasal root; microstomia; cleft palate; occasional cleft lip; micrognathia;

Growth: short stature;

Ocular: iris, choroid, retina, and/or optic nerve coloboma; microphthalmia;

Auditory: Mondini anomaly; semicircular canal hypoplasia;

Cardiac: heart anomalies, often conotruncal, but also endocardial cushion defect;

Skeletal: short neck; scoliosis;

Genital: small phallus in males; cryptorchidism; hypospadias;

Other: occasional anal anomalies, occasional renal anomalies; tracheoesophageal fistula has been reported in a few cases.

Natural History: Birthweight is often slightly low, and postnatal growth is slow resulting in progressive short stature. All developmental milestones are delayed and language and speech are particularly impaired. The cognitive delays are static, but may be severe in some cases.

Treatment Prognosis: Variable, depending on the severity of the cognitive impairment. Surgically resolving the choanal atresia often fails because it is difficult to maintain nasal patency. Children with CHARGE tend to be chronic mouth breathers.

Differential Diagnosis: Because the CHARGE symptoms are common in other syndromes and CHARGE is considered to be etiologically heterogeneous, the diagnosis of CHARGE should not rule out a syndromic diagnosis, as well. For example, children with **velo-cardio-facial syndrome** have been reported to have many or all of the CHARGE features. Other disorders with overlapping phenotypes include **cat eye syndrome,** VATER association, and a number of chromosomal syndromes, including trisomy 13, and del (4p) (Wolf-Hirschhorn syndrome).

Cleidocranial Dysplasia

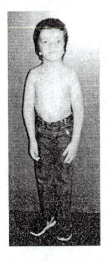
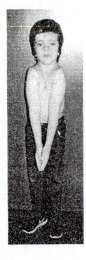
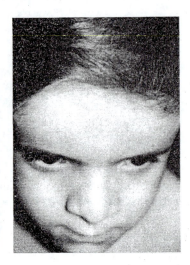

Cleidocranial dysplasia: Absence of the clavicles in a 5 year old boy with cleidocranial dysplasia permitting him to adduct his shoulders. Note the broad forehead (right).

Also Known As: Cleidocranial dysostosis.

Cleidocranial dysplasia is a distinctive syndrome that causes distinctive craniofacial and skeletal abnormalities. These abnormalities make the diagnosis relatively easy in cases with obvious expressions of the disorder. The population prevalence of the syndrome is not known, but hundreds of cases have been described in the medical literature.

Major System(s) Affected: Craniofacial; dental; skeletal; growth, limbs.

Etiology: Autosomal dominant mode of inheritance. The cause of the disorder is thought to be a deletion at 6p21.

Quick Clues: The prominent, broad, often bifid forehead associated with very narrow shoulders is a clear indication of cleidocranial dysplasia.

Hearing Disorders: Conductive hearing loss is a common finding, caused by minor anomalies of the ossicles and mastoid bone. The hearing loss is typically static.

Speech Disorders: Articulation disorders are common in cleidocranial dysplasia. In some cases, there are compensatory substitutions secondary to cleft palate and velopharyngeal insufficiency. However, in the majority of cases, the articulation disorder is related to dental spacing, malocclusions, and missing teeth. The errors are obligatory in nature.

Feeding Disorders: Feeding disorders are not common in cleidocranial dysplasia. Cleft palate is an infrequent finding in the syndrome but can complicate early attempts at feeding. In later life, delayed eruption of the primary and secondary teeth is common and can cause some problems with masticating certain types of food.

Voice Disorders: Voice is typically normal in cleidocranial dysplasia.

Resonance Disorders: Resonance may be hypernasal in cases with cleft palate, but is otherwise normal.

Language Disorders: Language and cognitive development are typically normal.

Other Clinical Features:

Craniofacial: Broad forehead, often with bilateral prominence of the frontal bone related to a patent metopic suture; macrocephaly, brachycephaly; late closure of the cranial sutures; large foramen magnum; occasional cleft palate; occasional mild hypertelorism; Class III malocclusion (relative prognathism);

Dental: delayed eruption of both the primary and secondary teeth; overretained primary dentition with root resorption; supernumerary secondary teeth;

Skeletal: absent or hypoplastic clavicles; narrow chest; short ribs; spina bifida occulta; reduced pelvic diameter;

Growth: relatively short stature;

Limbs: brachydactyly, joint laxity.

Natural History: At birth, unless the absence of the clavicles is obvious, the diagnosis can be difficult as babies look relatively normal. As the cranium and brain begin to grow, the delayed ossification of the cranium and resulting widely patent cranial sutures cause significant distortion of the skull. The head is large, the forehead tall, sometimes with bilateral prominences. The sutures eventually close. Some clinicians have suggested that children with cleidocranial dysplasia wear helmets to protect their brains from injury, but there have not been documented cases of brain trauma related to delayed ossification, possibly because the sutures do have a fibrous connection. As ossification of the cranium occurs, skull shape becomes more normal. Delayed dental eruption is particularly noticeable in the secondary dentition, because the primary teeth are often overretained so that the teeth appear very small with severe dental spacing. In females, the reduced pelvic diameter makes normal childbirth difficult so that Caesarean section is necessary.

Treatment Prognosis: The anomalies in cleidocranial dysplasia are not particularly debilitating. Absence of the clavicles does not cause any particular problems and the cranial anomalies resolve with time.

Differential Diagnosis: The association of cranial and clavicular anomalies in cleidocranial dysplasia is essentially unique.

Cockayne Syndrome

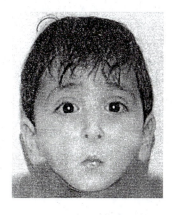

Cockayne syndrome: Note the triangular face with lack of subcutaneous fat in the cheeks.

Also Known As: Cockayne syndrome, type I; Cockayne syndrome, type A.

Cockayne syndrome is a rare but distinct syndrome of premature senility, early death, short stature, and deterioration of the central nervous system. Since its delineation, several subtypes have been identified with genetic etiologies different from the originally described phenotype. The "classic" Cockayne syndrome is now referred to as type I, or type A, by some clinicians. Two additional subtypes (II and III) have also been recognized.

Major System(s) Affected: Central nervous system; growth; skin; craniofacial; ocular; skeletal; cardiopulmonary, auditory; vascular.

Etiology: Autosomal recessive inheritance. The gene is thought to be located on chromosome 5.

Quick Clues: Short stature associated with the appearance of disproportionately long limbs and large hands is an initial clue to the diagnosis of Cockayne syndrome. Later in childhood, deterioration of cognitive functioning and premature senility (with the appearance of rapid aging) are strong indications.

Hearing Disorders: Hearing is initially normal, but with the onset

43

of neurologic deterioration, there is perceptual (central) hearing impairment.

Speech Disorders: Early speech development and production are often normal through toddler years. Then speech begins to deteriorate, and dysarthria is a common symptom. Eventually, speech deteriorates to the point of unintelligibility.

Feeding Disorders: Early feeding is normal. When neurologic deterioration begins, feeding may become disordered in a manner similar to that seen in geriatric patients.

Voice Disorders: Voice is high pitched.

Resonance Disorders: Resonance is initially normal, but with the onset of dysarthria, hypernasality may become pronounced.

Language Disorders: Language development is normal in its earliest stages, but during childhood, there is deterioration of all cognitive skills, including language.

Other Clinical Features:

Central nervous system: Progressive cognitive impairment; dementia; demyelination;

Growth: short stature;

Skin: photosensitivity; premature aging; pigmentary changes;

Craniofacial: microcephaly; deep set eyes; relative prognathism;

Ocular: retinal degeneration; retinal pigmentation anomalies; corneal degeneration;

Skeletal: limbs are disproportionately long; large hands and feet; joint contractures;

Cardiopulmonary: hypertension;

Auditory: central deafness;

Vascular: progressive atherosclerosis.

Natural History: Early development after birth may seem relatively normal until one to two years of age. Progressive cerebellar ataxia, choreoathetosis, and eventual blindness are inevitable; early death occurs following the precipitously downhill neurologic course.

Treatment Prognosis: Poor.

Differential Diagnosis: Premature senility is a key feature of progeria, but without the same neurologic sequelae. **Bloom syndrome** has similar degenerative skin findings. Progressive neurologic, skin, and visual impairment occur in **Refsum syndrome,** but without the growth abnormality.

Cockayne Syndrome, Type II

Also Known As: Cockayne syndrome, type B.

Cockayne syndrome, type II, is differentiated from type I by the age of onset and progression. The symptoms in Cockayne syndrome, type II, are similar to those of type I, but the expression of the syndrome is congenital, rather than an onset of two to four years of age, as seen in type I. Individuals with Cockayne syndrome, type II, are of low birth weight and grow very little, remaining very small and severely impaired. Although familial cases have not occurred, the gene is expressed in an autosomal dominant manner (i.e., only one mutant copy of the gene pair is required to express the syndrome).

Major System(s) Affected: Central nervous system; growth; skin.

Etiology: Autosomal dominant expression. The gene, *ERCC6*, has been mapped to 10q11.

Quick Clues: Low birthweight and severe cognitive impairment are not unique to this rare syndrome, but the lack of progression of growth and cognitive deterioration should lead to the consideration of the diagnosis. If it is noted that exposure to sunlight causes skin lesions, then the diagnosis becomes more likely.

Hearing Disorders: Central and sensorineural hearing impairment are probably common if not ubiquitous, but because of the severe impairment of the quality of life associated with this form of Cockayne syndrome, studies of the specific nature of hearing loss have not been performed or reported.

Speech Disorders: Speech does not develop.

Feeding Disorders: Feeding is severely impaired by neurologic degeneration. However, very poor growth is a primary feature of the syndrome and is not related to nutrition.

Voice Disorders: Voicing for communication does not develop.

Resonance Disorders: Speech does not develop.

Language Disorders: There is no language development.

Other Clinical Features:

> **Central nervous system:** severe mental retardation with progressive degeneration of neurologic function;
>
> **Growth:** very small stature;
>
> **Skin:** hypersensitivity to ultraviolet light.

Natural History: The syndrome is evident at birth and the neurologic findings worsen with age. Premature death is the rule following the progression of early onset senility.

Treatment Prognosis: Poor.

Differential Diagnosis: The neurologic findings are similar to those in **Cockayne syndrome, type I and type III** except that the disorder is obvious at birth. **Bloom syndrome** has similar skin findings without the neurological findings.

Cockayne Syndrome, Type III

Also Known As: Cockayne syndrome, type C.

Cockayne syndrome, type III, is marked by later onset and slower progression than in types I and II. Older patients have been described who are of normal stature.

Major System(s) Affected: Central nervous system; skin; growth; craniofacial; ocular; skeletal; cardiopulmonary.

Etiology: Autosomal recessive inheritance. The gene has not been mapped or identified.

Quick Clues: The association of an aged appearance with cognitive degeneration and disproportionately large hands and feet are strong clues to the diagnosis of Cockayne III.

Hearing Disorders: Perceptual and sensorineural hearing loss have both been observed.

Speech Disorders: Early speech development is often normal with subsequent deterioration after the onset of neurologic degeneration.

Feeding Disorders: Early feeding is normal. Dysphagia develops following the onset of neurologic deterioration.

Voice Disorders: Voice is normal.

Resonance Disorders: Resonance is normal, but hypernasality may present following the onset of neurologic degeneration.

Language Disorders: Early language development is normal, but deterioration occurs in childhood and adolescence in most cases.

Other Clinical Features:

> **Central nervous system:** neurologic deterioration; mental retardation; early dementia;
>
> **Skin:** sensitivity to sunlight; pigmentary anomalies; depletion of subcutaneous fat;
>
> **Growth:** small stature in most cases;
>
> **Craniofacial:** deep-set eyes; microcephaly; relative prognathism;

Ocular: retinal degeneration; optic atrophy; retinal pigmentation anomalies; corneal degeneration;

Skeletal: long limbs; comparatively large hands and feet;

Cardiopulmonary: hypertension.

Natural History: The progression is the same as type I, but the onset is slightly later and the progression less precipitous. However, the end-stage disease is similar.

Treatment Prognosis: Poor.

Differential Diagnosis: The phenotype is very similar to **Cockayne syndrome, type I.** The skin findings are similar to those seen in **Bloom syndrome.**

Coffin-Lowry Syndrome

Also Known As:

Coffin-Lowry syndrome was initially described in 1966 as a syndrome of severe mental retardation affecting only males. Subsequent observations of less severe manifestations of the disorder in female relatives has suggested X-linked dominant expression.

Major System(s) Affected:
Central nervous system; craniofacial; growth; skeletal; cardiac; renal; gastrointestinal; pulmonary.

Etiology: X-linked dominant mode of expression and inheritance. The gene has been mapped to Xp22.2-p22.1.

Quick Clues: The coarse facial appearance in Coffin-Lowry syndrome is distinctive, although other multiple anomaly disorders may also have facial features that could be described as "coarse," including the lysosomal storage diseases. However, unlike the majority of lysosomal storage diseases, infants with Coffin-Lowry syndrome show extremely poor cognitive development from birth, rather than at later onset.

Hearing Disorders: Sensorineural hearing loss has been observed in some cases, ranging from moderate to severe.

Speech Disorders: Affected males do not develop speech because of severe mental retardation.

Feeding Disorders: Early hypotonia may impair feeding and cause failure-to-thrive.

Voice Disorders: Voice is not used for speech in affected males, but hoarseness during vocalizations is common.

Resonance Disorders: Resonance disorders have not been observed, primarily because of the lack of speech development in affected males.

Language Disorders: Language is severely impaired, usually to the point of absence of language development in males. Female heterozygotes have mild to moderate language impairment.

Other Clinical Features:

Central nervous system: mental retardation, typically severe in males; hypotonia; hydrocephalus;

Craniofacial: coarse facial appearance; broad, flat nose; thick lips; anteverted nostrils; large ears; telecanthus; large mouth; prominent supraorbital ridge;

Growth: short stature; postnatal growth deficiency;

Musculoskeletal: cervical lordosis; kyphoscoliosis; pectus carinatum; flat feet; hyperextensible joints; tapered digits;

Cardiac: mitral valve regurgitation;

Renal: hydronephrosis;

Gastrointestinal: diverticulosis;

Pulmonary: restrictive pulmonary disease.

Natural History: Growth deficiency is of postnatal onset. Developmental impairment is evident very early. Postural changes, possibly secondary to hypotonia, lead to scoliosis, kyphosis, and cervical lordosis.

Treatment Prognosis: Very poor in males. Female heterozygotes typically have cognitive development ranging from normal to mildly impaired, although some are severely impaired.

Differential Diagnosis: The early facial appearance and hypotonia are somewhat reminiscent of **Williams syndrome,** but the absence of speech and language development soon differentiate the two diagnoses. The coarse facial features may also be mistaken for lysosomal storage diseases, which can be ruled out by metabolic testing.

Cowden Syndrome

Also Known As: Cowden disease; multiple hamartoma syndrome.

Cowden syndrome is a disorder that causes hamartomas, or nodular neoplasias, in multiple areas of the body, including the lips, tongue, oral gingiva, and palate. Hamartomatous growths also occur in glandular tissue, including the thyroid gland and the breasts.

Major System(s) Affected: Central nervous system; endocrine/glandular; skin; skeletal; craniofacial; gastrointestinal.

Etiology: Autosomal dominant inheritance. The gene, a tumor suppressor gene labeled *PTEN*, has been mapped to 10q23.3.

Quick Clues: The presence of multiple hamartomas on the lips and tongue are very distinctive.

Hearing Disorders: Sensorineural hearing loss is a low frequency anomaly in Cowden syndrome.

Speech Disorders: Articulation may be impaired in a number of ways related to the presence of oral hamartomas. Tongue placement can be altered because the surface of the tongue is not flat or smooth enough to make a broad contact with the alveolus, teeth, or palate. The lips may also have difficulty creating a tight seal because of multiple hamartomas. Distortions may also be caused by obligatory redirection of the airstream.

Feeding Disorders: The hamartomas occur later in life, usually in adolescence or early adult life, and are not present at birth. Early feeding is normal, and the hamartomas typically do not interfere with feeding in adult life, unless they require extensive surgical resection. Some of the hamartomas have been reported to develop into carcinomas requiring treatment.

Voice Disorders: Hoarseness is a common feature.

Resonance Disorders: Oral resonance may be muffled related to larger neoplasias in the oral cavity, especially posteriorly. Hypo-nasality may also occur related to adenoid enlargement.

Language Disorders: A small percentage of patients with Cowden syndrome may have mild cognitive impairment causing a language delay. In most cases, language is normal.

Other Clinical Features:

> **Central nervous system:** increased intracranial pressure; cognitive impairment in some cases; seizures; cerebellar anomalies; Chiari anomaly;

> **Endocrine/glandular:** hamartomas of the thyroid and breast;

> **Skin:** multiple hamartomas of the mucous membrane, particularly of the oral cavity; skin lesions on the face and limbs;

> **Skeletal:** pectus excavatum; scoliosis;

> **Craniofacial:** macrencephaly; oral hamartomas;

> **Gastrointestinal:** polypoid growth in the intestines;

Other: potential cancerous neoplasia of the brain, breast, skin, or kidneys.

Natural History: The hamartomas begin to develop in late childhood or early adolescence, and become larger and more numerous with age. Many of the neurological symptoms are related to later tumor growth and are not present in early life.

Treatment Prognosis: Symptomatic treatment may be valuable in removing particularly large growths that interfere with speech, but in some cases, the treatment may not improve function because the resection itself may leave excessive scar tissue. Additional growths may also appear in nearby tissues.

Differential Diagnosis: A number of syndromes may cause changes in the skin and mucous membrane of the oral cavity, including acanthosis nigricans, and Gardner syndrome, which has intestinal polyps. Proteus syndrome, the disorder expressed by the Elephant Man, results in many hamartomas, but they occur in regions other than the oral cavity and intestines.

Craniodiaphyseal Dysplasia

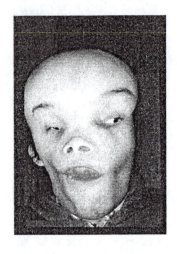

Craniodiaphyseal dysplasia: Severe craniofacial overgrowth associated with craniodiaphyseal dysplasia.

Also Known As: Leontiasis.

Craniodiaphyseal dysplasia is a rare syndrome of bony overgrowth of the craniofacial structures with associated abnormalities of the long bones. The overgrowth of the craniofacial skeleton is severe and may result in life-threatening compromise of the central nervous system and respiratory tract. The disorder was brought to public attention in the motion picture *Mask.*

Major System(s) Affected: Skeletal; craniofacial; central nervous system.

Etiology: The majority of cases that have been reported are of autosomal recessive etiology. However, autosomal dominant transmission of the syndrome has been observed. A gene has not been mapped or identified.

Quick Clues: Once the bony overgrowth has begun, the appearance of the face, cranium, and nose are unmistakeable.

Hearing Disorders: Mixed hearing loss is constant, beginning in early childhood, and is related to anomalies of the cranial bones, including the mastoid and ossicles. The hearing loss is typically progressive with eventual maximal or near maximal conductive loss and progressive neural loss related to compression of the cranial nerves.

Speech Disorders: Speech onset may be delayed. Bony overgrowth results in malocclusion and severe crowding of the oral cavity because of hyperostoses on the palate and jaws. Oral opening may be limited. There is severe articulatory impairment because of obligatory placement errors.

Feeding Disorders: In the neonatal period and infancy, feeding is not typically impaired. As the nasal cavity become increasingly more obstructed, there may be some difficulty with eating. Later in life, it may be necessary to shift diet to soft foods because of severe occlusal anomalies.

Voice Disorders: Voice disorders have not been reported or observed.

Resonance Disorders: Resonance becomes progressively more hyponasal with age, beginning in childhood. By adult life, there is total denasality. Oral resonance is also disordered because of maxillary and palatal skeletal overgrowth.

Language Disorders: Language may be normal in early life, although in some cases, there has been marked delay, especially of expressive language. With age and progressive compression of the brain, additional language impairment and cognitive impairment may occur.

Other Clinical Features:

Skeletal: diaphyseal dysplasia; absence of metaphyseal flaring of the long bones; sclerosis of mutliple skeletal components;

Craniofacial: severe overgrowth of the craniofacial skeleton leading to compromise of the nasal cavity, constriction of the cranial foramina, and compression of multiple nerves and blood vessels; orbital hypertelorism;

Central nervous system: compression of the cranial nerves; occasional cognitive impairment; increased intracranial pressure.

Natural History: The disorder is expressed shortly after birth and becomes obvious in childhood. The skeletal overgrowth reaches severe proportions quickly and compression of the cranial nerves becomes evident by the second decade of life. Respiratory obstruction also becomes progressively worse with severe obstructive sleep apnea caused by progressive narrowing of the upper airway because of skeletal overgrowth. The foramen magnum and other cranial foramina and fossae become obliterated or constricted and may result in sensory hearing loss, blindness, and early death. Increased intracranial pressure may result in progressive cognitive impairment. Obliteration of the sella turcica and pituitary gland results in lack of sexual maturation and short stature.

Treatment Prognosis: Poor. The disorder is relentlessly progressive and palliative treatments will have only temporary benefit.

Differential Diagnosis: Skeletal overgrowth of the craniofacial complex is common in **van Buchem disease,** osteosclerosis, **craniometaphyseal dysplasia,** and **frontometaphyseal dysplasia.** Craniodiaphyseal dysplasia differs from these other disorders in appearance of the long bones, which have absence of metaphyseal flaring.

Craniofrontonasal Syndrome

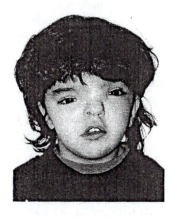

Craniofrontonasal dysplasia syndrome: Note severe hypertelorism and orbital asymmetry.

Also Known As: Craniofrontonasal dysplasia; craniofrontonasal dysostosis.

This X-linked syndrome results in a wide variety of craniofacial anomalies, including orbital hypertelorism, orbital dystopia, cleft palate, or cleft lip and palate. Hypertelorism is typically severe. The pattern of inheritance has been the subject of much speculation because females are more severely affected than males.

Major System(s) Affected: Craniofacial; integument; limbs; skeletal; genital; central nervous system.

Etiology: The disorder is inherited in an X-linked manner, but the mechanism of expression does not fit either dominant or recessive patterns. Inconsistent with X-linked dominant inheritance is the observation that the majority of familial cases observed and reported have been female-to-female transmission. The majority of known cases have been female, leading to initial speculation of male lethality by a possibly X-linked dominant trait. However, several male cases have been reported that are more mildly affected than females, an observation that is inconsistent with X-linked dominant transmission. However, no male-to-male cases have been observed, indicating that the gene is on the X chromosome. The gene has been mapped to Xp22.

Quick Clues: Hypertelorism accompanied by orbital dystopia (with the eyes at different vertical levels) is a common and distinctive finding in craniofrontonasal dysplasia syndrome.

Hearing Disorders: Conductive hearing loss secondary to chronic middle ear effusion is common and mixed loss has been observed in several cases.

Speech Disorders: Speech production is often affected by occlusal abnormalities resulting in obligatory distortions and substitutions. The presence of cleft palate or cleft lip and palate may result in compensatory articulation patterns.

Feeding Disorders: Feeding in infancy may be complicated by cleft palate, but is otherwise not impaired.

Voice Disorders: Hoarseness has been observed in some cases.

Resonance Disorders: Hypernasality secondary to cleft palate is common.

Language Disorders: Language impairment has been observed, as has cognitive impairment in some cases. However, language is often normal.

Other Clinical Features:

Craniofacial: orbital hypertelorism; orbital dystopia; cleft lip; cleft palate; low-set posteriorly rotated ears; broad nose with bifid tip;

Integument: coarse, wiry hair; longitudinal splitting of the fingernails;

Skeletal: Sprengel shoulder; pectus excavatum; clavicle anomalies;

Genital: hypospadias in males;

Central nervous system: occasional mental retardation; absence of the corpus callosum; learning disabilities.

Natural History: The disorder presents at birth and is nonprogressive.

Treatment Prognosis: Reconstructive surgery is indicated for resolution of structural anomalies.

The prognosis with current craniofacial surgery techniques is good.

Differential Diagnosis: Orbital hypertelorism or craniofacial anomalies in association with clavicle anomalies is seen in **cleidocranial dysplasia.** Isolated frontonasal dysplasia has very similar facial features, but no associated anomalies.

Craniometaphyseal Dysplasia

Also Known As:

Craniometaphyseal dysplasia occurs in two forms that are etiologically distinct, but clinically identical. The syndrome is marked by overgrowth of the craniofacial skeleton and generalized skeletal sclerosis and dysplasia of the long bones. Both the dominant and recessive forms are rare disorders.

Major System(s) Affected:
Craniofacial; skeletal; central nervous system.

Etiology: An autosomal dominant form has been mapped to 5p15.2-p14.1. The recessive form has not been mapped, nor the gene identified.

Quick Clues: Progressive thickening and prominence of the nasal root with elongation of the face accompanies the onset of a progressive mixed hearing loss in childhood.

Hearing Disorders: Progressive mixed hearing loss is common and is related to sclerosis of the temporal bone and mastoids. Hearing loss begins in childhood and progresses to severe levels later in adult life.

Speech Disorders: Obligatory articulation disorders include distortions secondary to malocclusion and anterior skeletal open-bite. The open-bite is caused by chronic open-mouth posture related to nasal obstruction from skeletal overgrowth. Eventually, cranial nerve compression may result in facial paresis and poor mobility of the oral musculature resulting in dysarthric speech production.

Feeding Disorders: Feeding is normal in infancy. After the beginning of craniofacial osteosclerosis, nasal obstruction ensues causing chronic mouth-breathing and some difficulty with large amounts of food being maintained in the mouth.

Voice Disorders: Voice disorders have not been reported.

Resonance Disorders: Resonance is hyponasal related to bony stenosis of the nasal cavity.

Language Disorders: Language development is normal.

Other Clinical Features:

Craniofacial: skeletal dysplasia and sclerosis; orbital hypertelorism; nasal stenosis; broad nasal root; facial paresis;

Skeletal: metaphyseal dysplasia; metaphyseal flaring;

Central nervous system: possible blindness secondary to optic nerve compression; occasional cognitive impairment.

Natural History: The onset of observable structural change in the face begins in late infancy or toddler years, usually with marked broadening of the nasal root. Progressive sclerosis proceeds unabated into adult life with resulting compression of cranial nerves II, VII, and VIII.

Treatment Prognosis: Palliative treatment has only temporary effects because the bone growth continues throughout life.

Differential Diagnosis: There are a number of syndromes with progressive sclerotic growth of bone, including **van Buchem syndrome,** sclerosteosis, Pyle disease, **craniodiaphyseal dysplasia,** and **frontometaphyseal dysplasia.** The differential diagnosis is based on radiographic differences in the type of skeletal dysplasia and the bones affected.

Crouzon Syndrome

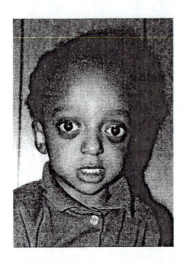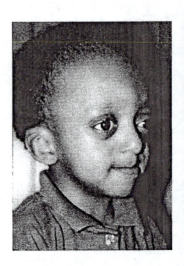

Crouzon syndrome: Four year old boy with Crouzon syndrome. Note the exorbitism and maxillary deficiency.

Also Known As: Craniofacial dysostosis.

Crouzon syndrome has been recognized as a genetic syndrome since its publication by Crouzon in 1912. In the past, many disorders with craniosynostosis were given the diagnostic label of Crouzon syndrome, probably inappropriately. Many new syndromes of craniosynostosis have been described since the delineation of Crouzon, and it is likely that many cases of **Pfeiffer syndrome, Jackson-Weiss syndrome,** and others have been mistakenly grouped together with Crouzon. The population prevalence of Crouzon syndrome is probably near 1:25,000 people. Crouzon differs from other syndromes of craniosynostosis in that all the findings are limited to the craniofacial skeleton.

Major System(s) Affected: Craniofacial

Etiology: Crouzon syndrome is caused by mutation of a single gene, *FGFR2* (fibroblast growth factor receptor 2) located on the long arm of chromosome 10 at 10q26. Inheritance is autosomal dominant with variable expression.

Quick Clues: Bulging eyes and a Class III malocclusion are easily visible findings in Crouzon syndrome and may be accompanied by an abnormal head shape.

Hearing Disorders: Conductive hearing loss is common, usually mild, and occasionally moderate. Probably more than half of individuals with Crouzon syndrome have hearing loss. Stenotic ear canals have been implicated, but chronic middle ear disease and ossicular anomalies may also be found.

Speech Disorders: Articulation disorders are very common, marked by obligatory distortions related to malocclusion, especially Class III maxillary retrusions and anterior skeletal open-bites, which are common in the syndrome. Resonance may also be hyponasal related to a small nasopharynx and nasal cavity. Cleft palate is a rare finding in the syndrome and is unlikely to cause significant hypernasality because of the reduced size of the nasopharynx.

Feeding Disorders: Upper airway obstruction and possible choanal atresia will result in failure-to-thrive because infants with Crouzon syndrome will strive to maintain respiration even at the expense of feeding. In such cases, the airway obstruction must be relieved.

Voice Disorders: Not a component of this syndrome.

Resonance Disorders: Hyponasality is common, related to reduced nasal cavity size and reduced nasopharyngeal volume.

Language Disorders: Language development is usually normal, unless there are sequelae of increased intracranial pressure.

Other Clinical Features: Maxillary hypoplasia, Class III malocclusion, occasional soft tissue hypertrophy of the hard palate, occasional cognitive impairment secondary to increased intracranial pressure and resulting brain damage; conductive hearing loss is common caused by both synostoses of the ossicles, and by reduced Eustachian tube function. Eustachian tube dysfunction is related to two factors: abnormal skull configuration caused by craniosynostosis results in an abnormal angulation and diameter of the tube; and the middle ear space is reduced in size and therefore is more easily filled with fluid. The clinical features of Crouzon syndrome are essentially limited to the craniofacial complex and the consequences of craniosynostosis. Abnormal skull shape, exorbitism (bulging eyes), malocclusion, dental crowding, ocular papilladema, and abnormal angulation of the ears are all secondary to the deforming effects of the skeletal growth abnormality of the cranial and facial bones. Hydrocephalus may occur, though less frequently than in **Apert syndrome** and **Pfeiffer syndrome.** Cleft palate has been reported in a small number of cases. Other findings, especially extracranial anomalies, are very rare and may be coincidental.

Natural History: Many infants with Crouzon syndrome appear normal at birth, though in some cases, the effects of synostosis are already apparent. With growth and age, progressive worsening of the midface deficiency becomes evident, becoming more obvious with the six year and pubertal growth spurts. If there is increasing intracranial pressure, there may be some neurologic deterioration, preceded by headaches, ataxia, or other psychomotor symptoms. The majority of patients with Crouzon syndrome have normal intellect and

development if the craniosynostosis is surgically corrected early in life (the optimal time being in infancy).

Treatment Prognosis: The prognosis for normal cognitive development is excellent, especially if craniectomy or cranial reconstruction is accomplished early in life. Children with Crouzon syndrome should be continuously checked for increased intracranial pressure until brain growth is complete. Obligatory articulation errors are related to skeletal anomalies which cause malocclusions. Therefore, resolution of the anterior sound distortions in Crouzon syndrome would not be expected until after correction of the occlusal anomalies by orthognathic surgery or midface advancement.

Differential Diagnosis: There are a number of syndromes that have craniosynostosis as a primary finding, including **Apert** and **Jackson-Weiss syndromes,** which are caused by a different mutation in the same *FGFR2* gene which causes Crouzon syndrome. Crouzon syndrome may be distinguished from other syndromes of craniosynostosis by the absence of limb anomalies and the better cognitive prognosis.

Cryptophthalmos Syndrome

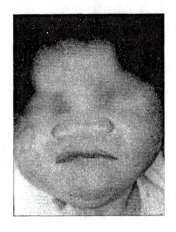

Cryptophthalmos syndrome: Note the absence of palpebral openings and the extension of hair onto the lateral aspects of the forehead.

Also Known As: Fraser syndrome; cryptophthalmos-syndactyly syndrome.

This distinctive syndrome involves cryptophthalmos (meaning "hidden eyes"). The syndrome's identifying characteristic is absence of palpebral fissures, but the eyes may be normal underneath a skin covering in some cases.

Major System(s) Affected: Ocular; craniofacial; limbs; gastrointestinal; genitourinary; central nervous system.

Etiology: Autosomal recessive inheritance. The gene has not been mapped or identified.

Quick Clues: The eye malformations in cryptophthalmos are unmistakable, but the association of a projection of hair near the orbit is essentially pathognomonic of the syndrome.

Hearing Disorders: Conductive hearing loss secondary to ossicular malformations is common. The external ear canal may also be stenotic.

Speech Disorders: Speech is delayed in most cases secondary to cognitive impairment. Articulation may also be impaired by compensatory articulation patterns in cases with cleft palate or cleft lip and palate (approximately 10%).

Feeding Disorders: Infant feeding may be compromised by respiratory distress secondary to laryngeal stenosis. Cleft palate may further complicate feeding.

Voice Disorders: Voice disorders have not been reported or observed.

Resonance Disorders: Hypernasal resonance may occur in patients with cleft palate.

Language Disorders: Language delay and impairment are common because of the frequency of cognitive impairment in the syndrome.

Other Clinical Features:

>**Ocular:** cryptophthalmos; eyelid coloboma; dermoid cysts; absent lens; corneal opacity; absent lacrimal glands;

Craniofacial: craniofacial asymmetry; hypertelorism; auricular anomalies; low-set ears; stenotic external auditory meatus; cleft palate with or without cleft lip; bifid nose or nasal tip; low anterior hair line; projection of hair on the face near the eyes;

Limbs: syndactyly;

Gastrointestinal: umbilical hernia; omphalocele; abnormal placement of umbilicus;

Genitourinary: renal anomalies; clitoral enlargement; malformed fallopian tubes; bicornate uterus; small male genitalia; hypospadias; cryptorchidism;

Central nervous system: cognitive impairment; encephalocele; Dandy-Walker anomaly.

Natural History: Some affected infants are stillborn or die shortly after birth. Blindness is typical, but sight has been restored by surgical means in some cases. Ambiguity of the genitalia has been seen and may result in ambiguous gender identity.

Treatment Prognosis: Overall prognosis is dependent on the degree of cognitive impairment.

Differential Diagnosis: There are no syndromes with significant phenotypic overlap with cryptophthalmos syndrome.

Cytomegalovirus Embryopathy

Also Known As: CMV embryopathy; fetal CMV syndrome.

Viral infections may have teratogenic influences if the virus is transplacental. The expression of this syndrome is dependent on the timing of the infection. An expansive phenotype is present when the infection is contracted within the first trimester. CMV is a large cell virus in the herpes virus group. Maternal infections are often undetected and the virus is ubiquitous in the general population.

Major System(s) Affected: Ocular; central nervous system; viscera.

Etiology: Cytomegalovirus infection (teratogenic).

Quick Clues: The presence of congenital cataracts in association with seizures and sensorineural hearing loss is indicative of CMV embryopathy.

Hearing Disorders: Bilateral congenital sensorineural hearing loss, typically profound or total, is the norm.

Speech Disorders: In the most severe cases, speech does not develop because of severe mental retardation. In milder cases, speech is affected by congenital deafness or profound hearing loss.

Feeding Disorders: In the most severe cases, severe neurological symptoms and hypotonia result in early failure to thrive.

Voice Disorders: Specific voice impairments have not been noted.

Resonance Disorders: Resonance may be impaired secondary to severe neurologic impairment in the most severe cases.

Language Disorders: In the most severe cases, expressive language may not develop, and receptive language may be severely impaired. In milder cases, language skills may be within the normal range.

Other Clinical Features:

Ocular: congenital cataracts; corneal opacification;

Central nervous system: primary microcephaly; cognitive impairment; seizures; intracranial calcifications; spasticity;

Viscera: hepatosplenomegaly; jaundice.

Natural History: The anomalies associated with CMV embryopathy are all present at birth and do not progress.

Treatment Prognosis: The prognosis for treatment is dependent on the severity of central nervous system impairment, when present. In the most severe cases, the prognosis for improvement and response to treatment is extremely poor.

Differential Diagnosis: Congenital cataracts are also caused by the teratogenic effects of cytomegalovirus. Corneal opacification is found in **Harboyan syndrome,** but without the central nervous system impairment seen in **rubella embryopathy.**

de Lange Syndrome

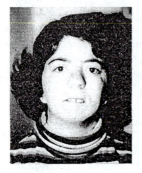
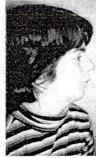

De Lange Syndrome: Facial appearance of an adolescent with de Lange syndrome with minor limb reduction anomalies, including shortening of the fifth fingers bilaterally.

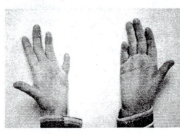
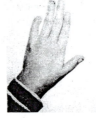
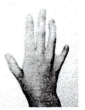

Also Known As: Cornelia de Lange syndrome; Brachmann-de Lange syndrome.

De Lange syndrome is a distinctive syndrome of mental retardation and small stature that is easily recognized and one of the more common multiple anomaly disorders associated with severe cognitive impairment. The population prevalence of de Lange syndrome is probably between 1:10,000 and 1:15,000. There is marked variability of expression.

Major System(s) Affected: Central nervous system; growth; limbs; craniofacial; integument; dental; musculoskeletal; cardiac; gastrointestinal; hematologic; genitals.

Etiology: The very large majority of de Lange cases are sporadic, but an autosomal dominant mode of expression and inheritance has been suggested, based on a small number of vertical pedigree transmissions. Trisomy of 3q26.3 has been found in a number of cases, but not all, and a single gene responsible for the syndrome located at 3q26.3 is possible, if not likely.

Quick Clues: The presence of synophrys (often comically referred to as a "unibrow") in association with microcephaly and developmental delay is an easily observable and distinctive feature of de Lange syndrome. The presence of limb reduction anomalies would further confirm the diagnosis.

Hearing Disorders: Hearing loss is probably underreported in de Lange syndrome, in part because the frequency of severe retardation and early death are so common. Both conductive and sensorineural hearing loss may occur in the syndrome. Conductive loss is secondary to chronic middle ear disease and effusion, sometimes related to cleft palate. Sensorineural hearing loss is variable, from mild to severe, and usually bilateral.

Speech Disorders: A high percentage of patients with de Lange syndrome are severely retarded and do not develop speech at all. However, more mildly affected cases have been recognized, and even though IQ does approach normal values, speech development is more severely impaired than other cognitive skills, and the onset of speech is severely delayed. Articulation is frequently impaired by a combination of factors, including severe malocclusion problems (micrognathia and Class II malocclusion) and compensatory substitutions related to cleft palate. Retromicrognathia (the lower jaw is both retruded and small) results in severe tongue backing and articulation impairment.

Feeding Disorders: Early feeding problems are very common in de Lange syndrome with failure-to-thrive a nearly consistent finding. The early feeding disorders are multifactorial in nature, contributed to by upper airway obstruction (micrognathia), dystonia and opisthotonic posture, esophageal stenosis, heart malformations, diaphragmatic hernia, and gastroesophageal reflux.

Voice Disorders: Hoarseness is common and may be detected in the early crying of babies with de Lange syndrome. The cry is often low pitched, as well.

Resonance Disorders: Both hypernasality and hyponasality may be observed. Hypernasality is common in the individuals with de Lange syndrome who have cleft palate. Hyponasality may occur in some cases because the nasal capsule is smaller than normal. Abnormal oral resonance is also common because of severe retro-micrognathia that causes the tongue to fall posteriorly in the oropharynx and hypopharynx producing a muffling of oral resonance.

Language Disorders: Language is often more severely impaired than would be expected in relation to the degree of cognitive impairment. In cases with severe cognitive impairment, expressive language rarely develops. In cases with less severe cognitive impairment, expressive language is typically more severely impaired than receptive language, and failure to develop expressive language is observed even in cases with moderate retardation. Because there is often limb reduction and absence of multiple digits in de Lange syndrome, signing may not be possible.

Other Clinical Features:

Central nervous system: Mental retardation; hyperto-
nia; opisthotonic posture; seizures;

Growth: small stature; low birthweight;

Limbs: limb reduction (phocomelia); missing digits, shortening of the forearms; absent tibia; bifurcate femur; low-set thumbs;

Craniofacial: thin upper lip; downturned oral commissures; retro-micrognathia; low-set posteriorly rotated ears; minor external ear anomalies; microcephaly;

Integument: hirsutism; synophrys; arched and flared eyebrows; hair growth on forehead and down the neck; cutis marmorata; multiple deeply pigmented nevi;

Dental: small teeth; dental spacing;

Musculoskeletal: limited joint mobility; delayed skeletal maturation;

Cardiac: heart anomalies (VSD, ASD, hypoplastic left ventricle);

Gastrointestinal: diaphragmatic hernia; esophageal/

pyloric stenosis; duplication of the colon; Meckel's diverticulum; gastroesophageal reflux;

Hematologic: thrombocytopenia;

Genitourinary: hypoplastic kidneys; cryptorchidism and hypospadias in males; bicornate uterus in females.

Natural History: Developmental milestones are globally delayed, but the onset of speech and language is far more severely impaired and rarely becomes commensurate with overall development. Life expectancy is shortened in many cases. Many infants develop pneumonias and other respiratory disorders with failure-to-thrive, with many succumbing in the neonatal period.

Treatment Prognosis: Variable, ranging from fair to poor in many areas, but typically poor in relation to expressive language and speech. A high percentage of individuals with de Lange syndrome are institutionalized.

Differential Diagnosis: The coarse facial appearance associated with mental retardation seen in de Lange syndrome may have some similarities to Coffin-Siris syndrome. However, the clinical manifestations of de Lange syndrome are very distinctive and diagnosis is not difficult.

Down Syndrome

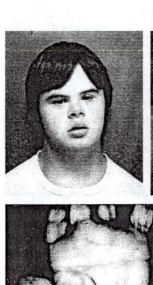

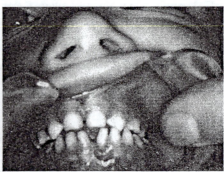

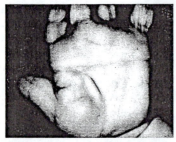

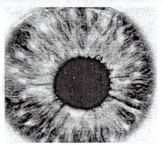

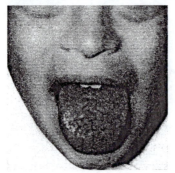

Down syndrome (trisomy 21):
Characteristic manifestations of
Down syndrome, including Brushfield
spots of the iris (lower right),
transverse palmar crease (middle
left), small teeth (upper right), and
large grooved tongue (lower left).

Also Known As: Trisomy 21.

Down syndrome is probably the most frequently occurring multiple anomaly disorder in humans with a population prevalence of approximately 1:1,000 people, although estimates vary somewhat. The syndrome was probably first described by Séguin in 1846, 20 years before John Langdon Down developed his theory of ethnic traits and their effect on intellect. Down coined the term "mongoloid idiot," clearly showing his racial bias in his 1866 treatise. As a result, his name has become eponymous with the syndrome. The presence of an extra chromosome as the cause of Down syndrome was not discovered until 1959. Although 95% of individuals with Down syndrome have a complete trisomy of chromosome 21, it is now understood that only a small segment of chromosome 21 at 21q22.3 is responsible for the majority of the phenotype.

Major system(s) affected: Central nervous system; craniofacial; growth; cardiac; gastrointestinal; limbs; ocular; hematologic.

Etiology: In 95% of cases, karyotype reveals an extra complete chromosome 21. In the balance of cases, the phenotype is caused by an unbalanced translocation or mosaicism. It has recently been discovered that only a portion of the genetic material on chromosome 21 is responsible for the majority of the Down syndrome phenotype. A "Down critical region" has been isolated to 21q22.3. Individuals with Down syndrome are sterile.

Quick Clues: The facial appearance of Down syndrome is distinctive and there is little chance of confusing another multiple anomaly disorder with the familiar facial expression of Down. However, individuals with a mosaic form of Down syndrome may be less obvious to the inexperienced clinician. Although the transverse palmar crease (or "simian crease") has gained some attention as a physical marker for Down syndrome, such dermatoglyphic markings are so common among the general population and among other multiple anomaly syndromes that it is essentially useless as a clinical identifier. Brushfield spots in the eyes, macroglossia, small teeth, small ears, and the Down habitus may be more informative at the level of casual inspection.

Hearing Disorders: Conductive, mixed, and sensorineural hearing loss have all been documented in individuals with Down syndrome. It is probable that the majority of hearing loss in individuals with Down syndrome is conductive secondary to chronic middle ear disease. Serous otitis and middle ear effusion are common in Down syndrome because of abnormal craniofacial anatomy, reduced immune function, decreased volume and abnormal angulation of the Eustachian tube. Structural anomalies of the ossicles and the cochlea have been reported, including decreased length of the cochlea.

Speech Disorders: Speech is characterized by multiple obligatory distortions secondary to a combination of structural anomalies, including macroglossia, maxillary hypoplasia, malocclusion, and dental anomalies. However, there is an overriding neurological component that causes a slurred speech pattern, but speech rate is typically increased, rather than decreased as one might observe in dysarthria. Speech rhythm disorders are also common and stuttering is more common in Down syndrome than in the general population. There is typically poor phrasing and impaired prosody. Even in cases with minimal structural anomalies or in whom reconstructive surgery has been per-

formed for tongue reduction and malocclusion, the neurologic components persist. Abnormalities of tongue movement are mostly related to motor control problems emanating from the central nervous system rather than from structural abnormalities. Articulation is severely impaired and unintelligible in many, if not most, cases. Cleft palate, while not a common anomaly in Down syndrome, does occur with greater frequency than in the general population and may result in compensatory substitutions in addition to the other articulation impairments.

Feeding Disorders: Early feeding is impaired by hypotonia and is often complicated by cardiac anomalies and/or cleft palate.

Voice Disorders: Hoarseness is very common and the voice is often of low pitch for somatic size.

Resonance Disorders: Nasal and oral resonance are often disordered in Down syndrome. Hypernasal resonance is common in most cases with cleft palate or cleft lip and palate. Oral resonance is often impaired secondary to tonsillar hypertrophy. Enlarged lymphoid tissue is common in Down syndrome and often leads to upper airway obstruction. Oral resonance is muffled in such cases, yielding a "potato-in-the-mouth" resonance pattern. The neck is often short in Down syndrome, enhancing the muffled resonance pattern.

Language Disorders: Language is essentially always impaired in Down syndrome. Many children with Down syndrome socialize easily and adeptly, often engaging in verbal exchange with children and adults. However, their social skills are typically in excess of their cognitive abilities. As they grow older, it is obvious that language is almost always telegraphic with markedly reduced utterance length and the omission of major components of language. Language skills plateau in childhood and remain stagnant. Auditory memory is typically severely impaired, as is short-term memory.

Other Clinical Features:

Central nervous system: mental retardation; Alzheimer's disease; hypotonia; cerebellar and cerebral hypoplasia; occasional CNS neoplasias;

Craniofacial: brachycephaly, microcephaly; maxillary

hypoplasia; macroglossia; geographic tongue; small ears; overfolded helices; downturned oral commissures; epicanthal folds; upslanting palpebral fissures;

Growth: small stature; obesity;

Cardiac: various congenital heart anomalies, including endocardial cushion defect;

Gastrointestinal: duodenal stenosis or atresia; imperforate anus;

Limbs: brachydactyly; clinodactyly; transverse palmar crease; single flexion crease of the small fingers;

Ocular: Brushfield spots of the iris;

Hematologic: leukemia.

Natural History: Initial presentation is one of severe hypotonia and delayed psychomotor development. With growth and development, social skills develop more rapidly than cognitive skills. Language and speech development are usually severely impaired. There is some progression of psychomotor milestones through early childhood, but there is an eventual plateau with failure to progress. Many affected individuals develop Alzheimer's disease and premature senility. Average life span in Down syndrome is approximately 35 years.

Treatment Prognosis: In individuals with trisomy 21, the prognosis is typically poor for cognitive development. Patients with mosaicism may have borderline or low normal intellect, and some individuals with trisomy 21 may have borderline cognitive function, but the majority are significantly impaired with retardation ranging from mild to severe. However, even in higher functioning cases, there is still some plateau effect. Therefore, it is extremely important to aggressively treat children with Down syndrome early, including early speech and language therapy.

Differential Diagnosis: Down syndrome has a singular and distinctive phenotype.

Dyskeratosis Congenita

Also Known As: Zinsser-Cole-Engman syndrome.

This X-linked disorder involves the progressive growth of skin lesions, particularly on the oral mucosa. It is a progressive disorder with reduced life span because of progressive anemia and the development of malignant neoplasias. Mental deficiency and behavioral anomalies are also a part of the phenotype. An apparently autosomal recessive form, far less common, has also been reported.

Major System(s) Affected: Skin/integument; growth; central nervous system; auditory; gastrointestinal; skeletal; immunologic; hematologic; ocular; genitals.

Etiology: X-linked recessive inheritance. The gene has been mapped to Xq28. The gene has been labelled *DKC1*.

Quick Clues: The skin lesions on the oral mucosa are easily visible and should raise suspicion of the diagnosis of dyskeratosis congenita.

Hearing Disorders: Conductive, sensorineural, and mixed hearing loss have all been noted in dyskeratosis congenita. Erosion of the tympanic membrane from the skin lesions occurs in many cases.

Speech Disorders: Initial speech development may be normal, although it is often delayed in those cases with cognitive impairment (the majority of patients with dyskeratosis congenita). Once the oral mucosal lesions begin to appear, they may cause significant interference with articulation. Skin atrophy and scarring often occur leading to decreased oral sensation. The mucosal lesions may become infected and painful, further complicating speech production.

Feeding Disorders: Neonatal feeding disorders have not been noted or reported. In later life, oral feeding may be complicated by oral lesions, infections, and neoplasias. However, after the onset of the skin lesions, dysphagia may develop because of strictures in the digestive tract related to mucosal lesions or neoplasias. Gastrointestinal hemorrhage occurs from mucosal ulcerations.

Voice Disorders: Hoarseness secondary to laryngeal lesions is common.

Resonance Disorders: Resonance disorders are not common unless oral and pharyngeal lesions or neoplasias are large enough to interfere with pharyngeal or velopharyngeal function. Nasopharyngeal tumors have also been reported that may result in hyponasality.

Language Disorders: Language impairment is common in the more than 50% of individuals with this syndrome who are cognitively impaired. Mental retardation is a common manifestation of the syndrome.

Other Clinical Features:

Skin/integument: Areas of skin hyper/hypopigmentation; skin lesions (plaques) that result in atrophy and scarring; oral mucosa lesions; nail dystrophy;

Growth: small stature;

Central nervous system: cognitive impairment;

Auditory: sensorineural, conductive, or mixed hearing loss;

Gastrointestinal: ulcerative lesions in the intestines, rectum, and esophagus;

Skeletal: femoral head necrosis;

Immunologic: infections;

Hematologic: anemia; thrombocytopenia; pancytopenia;

Ocular: lacrimal duct obstruction;

Genitals: testicular atrophy;

Other: development of oral and anal malignant neoplasias; pancreatic cancer; Hodgkin's lymphoma.

Natural History: The onset of the growth of skin lesions occurs typically in childhood, generally by five years of age. Early death from neoplasias or anemia occurs frequently, often by the third decade of life, although some individuals live into the fifth and sixth decade. The lesions are progressive, and with age, the risk for anemia and cancer increases.

Treatment Prognosis: Fair. The disorder is progressive, but individual lesions can be treated successfully.

Differential Diagnosis: The skin lesions are similar to those seen in Fanconi pancytopenia, Rothmund-Thompson syndrome, and **Bloom syndrome,** but the natural history of this disorder differs from these other entities.

D

Dysosteosclerosis

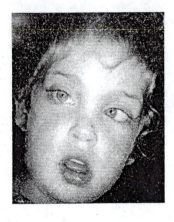

Dysosteosclerosis: Note the strabismus secondary to visual loss, and the flaccid facial appearance secondary to compression of cranial nerves.

Also Known As:

Dysosteosclerosis is a rare syndrome of advancing bone sclerosis that is significant with regard to communication impairment because of the possibility of compression of the cranial nerves. Effects on both speech and hearing have been observed, and in some rare cases, there has been progressive cognitive impairment.

Major System(s) Affected:
Growth; skeletal; craniofacial; neurological; dental.

Etiology:
Autosomal recessive inheritance. The gene has not yet been mapped or identified.

Hearing Disorders:
Otosclerosis is a common finding resulting in progressive hearing loss. The age of onset is earlier than otosclerosis in the general population.

Speech Disorders:
Speech development is typically normal, but if there is significant cranial nerve compression, facial paresis is a possible manifestation that can affect both articulation and rate of speech.

Feeding Disorders:
Early feeding is not problematic.

Voice Disorders:
Voice disorders have not been reported or observed.

Resonance Disorders: Resonance disorders have not been reported or observed.

Language Disorders: Language development is normal in most cases, but may deteriorate in those cases with progressive cognitive impairment.

Other Clinical Features:

Growth: short stature;

Skeletal: progressive osteosclerosis; increased frequency of fractures; abnormal growth of the epiphyses, metaphyses, and diaphyses;

Craniofacial: sclerosis of the frontal bone and skull base; hyperostoses of the cranium; late closure of the anterior fontanel;

Neurological: cranial nerve compression; facial paresis; optic nerve compression;

Dental: delayed eruption of permanent dentition; small teeth; deficient enamel.

Natural History: The skeletal anomalies are present at birth, but become progressively worse with age. The onset of cranial nerve compression may begin in early childhood. The onset of otosclerosis is earlier than is typical.

Treatment Prognosis: The osteosclerosis that results in cranial nerve compression cannot be resolved with surgery. Therefore, in the most severe cases, the prognosis is poor.

Differential Diagnosis: There are a number of other syndromes with progressive osteosclerosis, including **van Buchem syndrome** and sclerosteosis, neither of which has short stature as a clinical finding. Robinow syndrome has short stature as a common finding along with mild osteosclerosis, but the facies in Robinow is distinctive and dysmorphic, which is not the case in dysosteosclerosis.

Edwards Syndrome

Also Known As: Pigmentary retinopathy, diabetes mellitus, hypogonadism, mental retardation, and sensorineural hearing loss.

This syndrome resembles **Alström syndrome,** except that mental retardation is one of the major findings in Edwards syndrome that is not present in **Alström.** The label "Edwards syndrome" should not be confused with the same nosologic identification for trisomy 18. These are separate and distinct disorders and, unlike Edwards syndrome, trisomy 18 is typically incompatible with life.

Major System(s) Affected: Ocular; central nervous system; integument; genitourinary; endocrine.

Etiology: Autosomal recessive inheritance. The gene has not been mapped or identified.

Quick Clues: The association of nystagmus with short stature and sensorineural hearing loss are clues to the diagnosis of this rare condition.

Hearing Disorders: Bilateral sensorineural hearing loss typically has its onset in childhood, before puberty, and slowly progresses to a moderate to severe impairment.

Speech Disorders: Speech is delayed in nearly all cases, and in the most severe cases, there may be severe delay in the onset of speech milestones.

Feeding Disorders: Feeding is not impaired.

Voice Disorders: Voice is high pitched.

Resonance Disorders: Resonance is not impaired.

Language Disorders: Language is uniformly impaired consistent with the degree of cognitive deficiency.

Other Clinical Features:

> **Ocular:** nystagmus; photophobia; pigment anomalies of the retina;

> **Central nervous system:** cognitive deficiency, typically mild to moderate;

Integument: acanthosis nigricans;

Genitourinary: hypogonadism;

Endocrine: diabetes mellitus; obesity; short stature.

Natural History: The onset of visual impairment occurs typically in the first year of life, hearing loss occurring somewhat later. Development tal delay and cognitive impairment are congenital.

Treatment Prognosis: The hearing impairment progresses slowly and is therefore amenable to amplification as long as there is careful follow-up.

Differential Diagnosis: Other than the cognitive impairment, Edwards syndrome is very similar to **Alström syndrome.**

EEC Syndrome

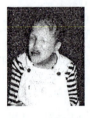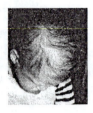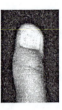

EEC syndrome: (left to right) An eight-year-old girl with EEC syndrome showing bilateral cleft lip and palate, ectrodactyly of the feet and hands, sparse scalp hair, and a hypoplastic nail on the thumb.

Also Known As: Ectrodactyly, ectodermal dysplasia, and clefting.

EEC is an easily recognized multiple anomaly disorder because of the combination of clefting, hand and foot anomalies, dental anomalies, and abnormal hair. Because all these malformations are easy to see by even casual examination, EEC is a syndrome that most clinicians have little trouble recognizing. EEC is also one of a number of syndromes with mixing of cleft type within a single pedigree. In other words, some individuals in the same family may have cleft palate, while others have cleft lip and palate. The mixing of cleft types within the same family only occurs in syndromic cleft-ing. There is marked variability of expression.

Major System(s) Affected: Craniofacial; limbs; integument; ocular; dental; genitourinary; central nervous system.

Etiology: Autosomal dominant inheritance. The gene has been mapped to 7q11.2-q21.3.

Quick Clues: One of the diagnostic hallmarks of the syndrome is ectrodactyly, often referred to as a "lobster claw" hand. Ectrodactyly is a relatively rare clinical finding outside of patients with EEC. The scalp hair in EEC is also distinctive with the hair often being of light color and appearing brittle, much like a wig made of artificial hair.

Hearing Disorders: Conductive hearing loss occurs secondary to middle ear effusion and also secondary to ossicular anomalies. Sensorineural hearing loss has also been reported. Conductive hearing loss is often moderate and more severe in low frequencies.

Speech Disorders: Articulation distortions are common in the syndrome because of large gaps caused by congenitally missing teeth and abnormally small and malformed teeth. Maxillary hypoplasia and Class III malocclusion also cause anterior obligatory distortions and lingual protrusion. Cleft palate or cleft lip and palate can also result in compensatory articulation patterns.

Feeding Disorders: Early feeding may be minimally complicated by cleft palate.

Voice Disorders: Hoarseness is common.

Resonance Disorders: Hypernasality secondary to cleft palate and resultant velopharyngeal insufficiency may occur. Choanal atresia has been reported as an infrequent finding and results in hyponasality.

Language Disorders: Language development is usually normal, but cognitive impairment and language delay occur as a low frequency anomaly (approximately 5 to 10% of cases). The author has had one patient who did not develop expressive language and was severely retarded.

Other Clinical Features:

>   **Craniofacial:** Cleft palate with or without cleft lip; maxillary hypoplasia; choanal atresia; microcephaly;
>
>   **Limbs:** ectrodactyly; cleft hands and feet; syndactyly; missing digits;
>
>   **Integument:** hypohydrosis; thin skin; very fair skin; very light, brittle hair; sparse hair; hypoplastic or absent nails; sparse eyelashes and eyebrows;
>
>   **Ocular:** sensitivity to light (photophobia); dacryocystitis; absent punctae; inflammation and infection of the eyelids;
>
>   **Dental:** missing teeth; malformed teeth; thin enamel;

Genitourinary: renal anomalies; ureter anomalies; hydronephrosis; hydroureter; cryptorchidism; hypospadias;

Central nervous system: cognitive impairment.

Natural History: The anomalies associated with EEC syndrome are present at birth and are nonprogressive. Hoarseness is related to hypohydrosis and lack of lubrication of the vocal cords. Maxillary hypoplasia is always present, but gets relatively more severe as the mandible grows in adolescence. By late teen years, midface deficiency is severe. In part, there is lack of vertical growth of the maxilla because of deficient alveolar bone, caused by missing teeth and small teeth with small roots.

Treatment Prognosis: In cases without cognitive impairment, the prognosis is good. Speech disorders can be treated as in other patients with clefts. Dentition can be restored with prosthetics or implants. There is no contraindication to maxillary surgery in late teen years.

Differential Diagnosis: Ectodermal dysplasia and clefting occur in AEC syndrome and Rapp-Hodgkin syndrome. However, neither of these syndromes has digit reduction or clefting of the hands and feet.

Ehlers-Danlos Syndrome, Type VI

Also Known As: EDS VI; Ehlers-Danlos, ocular form; keratoconus, keratoglobus, blue sclerae, loose ligaments, and hearing loss.

Ehlers-Danlos syndrome was first delineated as a single diagnostic entity involving joint and skin laxity, but it was subsequently recognized that there were multiple disorders under the umbrella of Ehlers-Danlos that were etiologically different and of variable phenotypes. Type VI is the form of Ehlers-Danlos that features hearing loss consistently.

Major System(s) Affected: Integument; ocular; cardiac; musculoskeletal; gastrointestinal; abdominal.

Etiology: Autosomal recessive inheritance. A mutation in the gene for lysyl hydroxylase, mapped to 1p36.3-p36.2, is likely.

Quick Clues: Severe joint laxity with loose and fragile skin are clues to the diagnosis of all the Ehlers-Danlos subtypes.

Hearing Disorders: Mixed hearing loss is most common with conductive components, consistent with otosclerosis in some cases.

Speech Disorders: Speech is typically normal.

Feeding Disorders: Feeding disorders have not been observed.

Voice Disorders: Voice disorders have not been observed or reported.

Resonance Disorders: Resonance is normal.

Language Disorders: Language development is normal.

Other Clinical Features:

> **Integument:** loose skin; chronic bruising of the skin;
>
> **Ocular:** microcornea; myopia; retinal detachment;
>
> **Cardiac:** mitral valve prolapse; aneurysms; carotid-cavernous fistula;

Musculoskeletal: scoliosis; kyphosis; joint hypermobility; joint dislocations; pes planus;

Gastrointestinal: diverticulosis; rupture of the colon;

Abdominal: inguinal hernia.

Natural History: Although all anomalies are related to connective tissue dysplasia that is present at birth, the problems appear to be progressive because the joints, ocular system, and middle ear structures tend to deteriorate with age.

Treatment Prognosis: The prognosis for individuals with Ehlers-Danlos, type VI is good, as it is for most individuals with connective tissue dysplasias. However, because of the risk of dissecting aortic aneurysm, careful medical follow-up is recommended.

Differential Diagnosis: Lax joints and loose skin occur in essentially all the subtypes of Ehlers-Danlos syndrome.

Escobar Syndrome

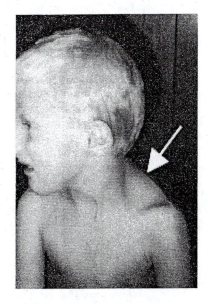

Escobar syndrome: Pterygium colli (arrow) in Escobar syndrome.

Also Known As: Pterygium syndrome; multiple pterygium syndrome; pterygium colli syndrome.

There is some confusion in the naming of this syndrome, and probably a number of different multiple anomaly disorders have come under the label of "multiple pterygium syndrome." This author prefers the label of Escobar syndrome in recognition of Victor Escobar's detailed delineation of the syndrome over two decades ago. The use of pterygium syndrome, multiple pterygium syndrome, or pterygium colli syndrome can be somewhat confusing in relation to other syndromes, including popliteal pterygium syndrome. Escobar syndrome is a distinct entity with distinctive differences from popliteal pterygium syndrome.

Major System(s) Affected: Growth; limbs; craniofacial; musculoskeletal; genital; cardiopulmonary; gastrointestinal.

Etiology: Autosomal recessive inheritance. The gene has not been mapped or identified.

Quick Clues: The presence of multiple pterygia is associated with only a few syndromes, including Escobar syndrome and popliteal pterygium syndrome. The pterygia in Escobar syndrome are easily noticed by even casual observation.

Hearing Disorders: Conductive hearing loss is common.

Speech Disorders: Articulation is impaired by a combination of factors. There is usually severe micrognathia with limited oral opening and restriction of mandibular range of motion. Cleft palate with or without cleft lip may add compensatory articulation patterns. Most common is severe tongue-backing related to the limited mandibular motion.

Feeding Disorders: Early feeding is often impaired by airway obstruction and glossoptosis.

Voice Disorders: Voice disorders have not been reported or observed.

Resonance Disorders: Both oral and nasal resonance disorders may occur. Hypernasality occurs secondary to cleft palate. Oral resonance is impaired by retropositioning of the mandible and tongue, causing a severely muffled oral resonance, which may assist in directing resonance through the nasal cavity because of limited oral opening.

Language Disorders: Language development is normal.

Other Clinical Features:

> **Growth:** small stature;
>
> **Limbs:** severe contractures of the fingers and toes; multiple joint contractures; rocker-bottom feet; syndactyly;
>
> **Craniofacial:** micrognathia; cleft palate with or without cleft lip; limited oral opening; low posterior hair line; downslanting palpebral fissures; downturned oral commissures;
>
> **Musculoskeletal:** multiple pterygia , including the neck, popliteal spaces, elbows; vertebral fusions; kyphoscoliosis; pectus carinatum; muscle hypoplasia;

Genital: cryptorchidism; small male genitals; absence of the labia majora; small clitoris;

Cardiopulmonary: pulmonary restriction; dilated aortic root; small heart;

Gastrointestinal: short ascending colon; absent appendix.

Natural History: The contractures are present at birth, but become progressively worse with growth. Muscle wasting follows.

Treatment Prognosis: The pterygia can not be surgically removed because vital nerves and vasculature are integrated within them. Oral management is also difficult because of persistent posterior pulling by the pterygia colli.

Differential Diagnosis: Multiple pterygia are also common in popliteal pterygium syndrome, but do not occur in the upper body. **Noonan syndrome** and **Turner syndrome** both have pterygia colli, but the heart and endocrine disorders distinguish these syndromes from Escobar syndrome.

Fabry Syndrome

Also Known As: Fabry disease; Anderson-Fabry disease; hereditary dystopic lipidosis.

Fabry syndrome has been a recognized clinical entity for over 100 years and is now understood to be a genetic inability to break down glycolipids, so that they are stored in some of the body's tissues, specifically the lysosomes of the skin, cornea, and smooth muscle. Dark nodular growths known as angiectases form in the skin, especially on the genitals, knees, umbilical area, buttocks, and mucous membranes.

Major System(s) Affected: Skin; ocular; renal; nervous system; cardiac.

Etiology: X-linked. The gene has been mapped to Xq22. The gene has been cloned and is labeled *GLA* and known to be approximately 12 kilobases in length.

Quick Clues: Dark pigmented lesions of the skin and swelling of the lips are easily noticeable and become progressively worse with age.

Hearing Disorders: High frequency sensorineural loss and diminished vestibular function are common findings.

Speech Disorders: Storage of glycolipids in the lips and oral mucosa may interfere with articulatory placement.

Feeding Disorders: Early feeding is normal. Feeding later in life may be impaired, following cerebrovascular event or strokes leading to dysphagia. Feeding may also be affected by airway obstruction caused by swelling of the upper and lower airway mucosal linings. Chronic diarrhea, nausea, and vomiting are common and may interrupt normal dietary habits.

Voice Disorders: Early voice is normal, but may eventually become hoarse secondary to storage of glycolipids in the laryngeal mucosa.

Resonance Disorders: Resonance may become hyponasal, related to growths and swelling of the nasal or nasopharyngeal mucosa.

Language Disorders: Language development is usually normal, but later in life cerebrovascular events may result in aphasia.

Other Clinical Features:

Skin: development of angiectases, or angiokeratomas (dark nodular lesions); lesions and swelling of the mucous membranes;

Ocular: surface corneal opacity; vascular lesions of the fundus;

Renal: renal failure;

Nervous system: chronic acroparesthesia; seizures; cerebrovascular events; chronic headaches; dizziness; hemiplegia;

Cardiac: angina; ECG abnormalities; septal hypertrophy.

Natural History: The skin lesions are first noted in late childhood, usually after 10 years of age, and then become progressively more numerous. The major debilitating symptom of the syndrome is chronic and intractable burning pain that also begins in childhood and may be brought on by external temperature shifts, exercise, or an illness with fever. Renal failure occurs somewhat later and is progressive. Life span is typically shortened to an average of approximately 45 years.

Treatment Prognosis: The disorder is progressive and related to a primary metabolic error. The long term prognosis is poor.

Differential Diagnosis: Syndromes with multiple dark skin lesions include **multiple lentigines syndrome** (LEOPARD syndrome), basal cell nevus syndrome, and Peutz-Jeghers syndrome. However, the lesions in these syndromes are qualitatively different from Fabry syndrome, and are easily distinguished by close examination.

Facio-oculo-acoustico-renal Syndrome

Also Known As: Holmes-Schepens syndrome; FOAR syndrome.

This rare syndrome has been reported in both relatives and single cases from unrelated families. In some ways, the syndrome bears a slight resemblance to **Stickler syndrome** and **Marshall syndrome** because of the association of congenital myopia, a depressed nasal root and epiphyseal dysplasia. However, this disorder has an autotomsal recessive pattern of inheritance and the hearing loss is more severe than found in **Stickler** or **Marshall syndromes.**

Major System(s) Affected: Craniofacial; ocular; musculoskeletal; central nervous system; abdominal.

Etiology: Autosomal recessive inheritance. The gene has not been mapped or identified.

Quick Clues: The combined facial characteristics of depressed nasal root, frontal bossing, and orbital hypertelorism are striking, but not necessarily unique to facio-oculo-acoustico-renal syndrome.

Hearing Disorders: Severe to profound sensorineural hearing loss. Vestibular abnormalities have not been reported.

Speech Disorders: Speech is likely to be delayed, primarily related to the severity of the hearing loss.

Feeding Disorders: Feeding disorders have not been observed.

Voice Disorders: Voice disorders have not been reported.

Resonance Disorders: Resonance is likely to be impaired by the hearing impairment.

Language Disorders: Language will be delayed and impaired by the severity of the hearing loss, but mild cognitive impairment is also possible.

Other Clinical Features:

Craniofacial: depressed nasal root; orbital hypertelorism; frontal bossing;

Ocular: myopia; cataracts; choroidal atrophy; retinal detachment;

Musculoskeletal: femoral epiphyseal dysplasia;

Central nervous system: mild cognitive impairment;

Abdominal: inguinal hernia; umbilical hernia.

Natural History: The visual impairments are progressive, and when congenital myopia is present, the disorder may progress to retinal detachment and blindness. The hearing loss is congenital.

Treatment Prognosis: The ocular anomalies may be treated by both preventive options and eventual surgery.

Differential Diagnosis: Stickler syndrome and Marshall syndrome have similar, but less severe, clinical features.

Facioscapulohumeral Muscular Dystrophy

Also Known As: Landouzy-Dejerine muscular dystrophy.

Facioscapulohumeral muscular dystrophy is one of the most common forms of myopathy. Only Duchenne muscular dystrophy and myotonic dystrophy are more common. When the onset of the disorder is early in childhood, there is a higher frequency of hearing loss. In cases with later onset, hearing loss is relatively uncommon. There is no particular correlation between the degree of muscle weakness and the extent of hearing loss.

Major System(s) Affected: Muscular; ocular; auditory; cardiopulmonary; skeletal.

Etiology: Autosomal dominant inheritance. The gene has been mapped to 4q35.

Quick Clues: Facial weakness results in a persistent mouth-open posture and the development of an anterior skeletal open-bite. Although similar findings are common in other neuromuscular diseases, the detection of facial and limb weakness will lead to appropriate referral for the possible diagnosis of a myopathy.

Hearing Disorders: Sensorineural hearing loss is common, especially in the early onset form. The hearing loss is sensory (cochlear), with normal nerve conduction to the brain.

Speech Disorders: Weakness of the facial muscles leads to secondary growth disturbance of the mandible and maxilla with vertical growth pattern, anterior skeletal open-bite, and increased lower face height. Malocclusion is common, and often presents as occlusion posteriorly on the molars, with the rest of the bite open. This leads to anterior lingual protrusion and obligatory distortions and substitutions for lingua-dental and lingua-alveolar sounds. Articulation may also be sluggish and slightly dysarthric.

Feeding Disorders: Early feeding is not typically problematic and, even with the onset of the muscle disease, swallowing is not impaired. However, chewing may be problematic because of the malocclusion.

Voice Disorders: Voice is typically normal, but mild breathiness may occur.

Resonance Disorders: Hypernasality relative to muscle weakness of the palate and pharynx is common.

Language Disorders: Language development is normal.

Other Clinical Features:

> **Muscular:** facial, trunk, and upper arm muscle weakness; leg weakness may occur later in life;

> **Ocular:** vascular anomalies of the retina; retinal detachment; macular degeneration;

> **Auditory:** sensorineural hearing loss;

> **Cardiopulmonary:** atrial tachycardia; cor pulmonale secondary to respiratory restriction and obstructive apnea; pulmonary restriction;

> **Skeletal:** secondary distortion and deformation of the skeleton, including scapular winging; flattening of the clavicles, and vertical facial growth pattern with steep mandibular plane angle.

Natural History: The obvious manifestations of the disorder may be recognized in childhood, including changes in facial structure, spontaneous onset of hypernasality, general facial weakness, and sensorineural hearing loss. The onset of weakness in the trunk and upper arms may not occur until many years later. Life expectancy may not be affected.

Treatment Prognosis: Hypernasality may be treated surgically or prosthetically, although surgical management must be approached carefully because of anesthesia risks. Dentofacial anomalies may also be treated with orthognathic surgery.

Differential Diagnosis: Facioscapulohumeral muscular dystrophy has similarities in terms of muscle weakness to other muscular dystrophies, but is a more benign form. Hypernasality may be seen in many other neuropathies, including **Steinert syndrome** (myotonic dystrophy), nemaline myopathy, and oculopharyngeal muscular dystrophy.

Fetal Alcohol Syndrome

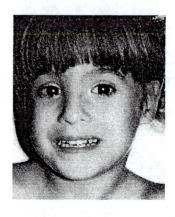

Fetal alcohol syndrome: Note the short palpebral fissures and thin upper lip associated with alcohol teratogenesis.

Also Known As: Fetal alcohol effects; ethyl alcohol embryopathy.

Although fetal alcohol syndrome did not become a well delineated diagnostic entity until the 1970s, the recognition of the teratogenic effects of alcohol had probably been understood for hundreds of years. Although clinicians are often taught to recognize the "typical" features of the teratogenic effects of ethanol, the reality is that the phenotype is highly variable because the expression of the disorder is dependent on a number of variables, including:

1. The amount of alcohol consumed by the mother.

2. The ability of the mother to metabolize the alcohol consumed before it reaches the placenta and developing embryo.

3. The stage of develoment of the embryo/fetus and the susceptibility of the particular tissues developing most vigorously at the time of alcohol consumption. For example, alcohol teratogenesis during the first trimester will result in structural anomalies, but in the last trimester the primary effect will be on the brain, which has active development in that trimester, whereas most organ systems and structures have already completed formation.

4. The duration of exposure to alcohol.

Debates about the amount of alcohol that might be "safe" to consume during pregnancy have not typically taken into account these four variables, in part because they cannot be properly assessed in individual cases in a systematic manner. The diagnosis of fetal alcohol syndrome is made based on a history of maternal alcohol consumption (paternal consumption is not teratogenic), so effects are assessed retrospectively in humans, and the history provided by alcoholic mothers may not be completely accurate. Although the teratogenic effects of alcohol can be assessed systematically in animals, the effects may not be entirely applicable to human development.

Major System(s) Affected:
Central nervous system; growth; cardiac; craniofacial; immune; ocular; genitourinary; integument; musculoskeletal; limbs.

Etiology: Maternal consumption of alcohol during pregnancy.

Quick Clues: The most obvious facial manifestations of fetal alcohol syndrome are small, close-set eyes and a thin upper lip and smooth philtrum, resulting in a poorly defined cupid's bow.

Hearing Disorders: Conductive hearing loss secondary to chronic middle ear effusion is common. Immune disorders are common in fetal alcohol syndrome, so that middle ear disease is both chronic and severe. External and middle ear anomalies may also occur resulting in more severe conductive hearing loss.

Speech Disorders: Onset of speech is delayed commensurate with the degree of cognitive impairment. Articulation is often impaired secondary to neurologically based discoordination. Dental spacing problems secondary to small teeth and bimaxillary protrusion with hypertrophic alveolar ridges may cause distortions. Anterior skeletal open-bite may occur secondary to hypotonia. Compensatory articulation patterns secondary to cleft palate and velopharyngeal insufficiency may also be found.

Feeding Disorders: Early failure-to-thrive is common secondary to hypotonia, irritability, airway obstruction, and micrognathia.

Voice Disorders: Hoarseness is common in fetal alcohol syndrome, in part because of vocal abuse in infancy from persistent vigorous crying.

Resonance Disorders: Hypernasal resonance secondary to velopharyngeal insufficiency is common in cases with cleft palate.

Language Disorders: Language impairment is essentially always present. Both receptive and expressive language are equally impaired, but unless cognitive impairment is severe, most individuals with fetal alcohol syndrome develop functional language.

Other Clinical Features:

> **Central nervous system:** mental retardation; learning disabilities (in milder cases); neonatal irritability; gray matter heterotopia;

> **Growth:** low birth weight; small stature;

> **Cardiac:** ventricular and atrial septal defects; tetralogy of Fallot; pulmonic stenosis; dextrocardia; right sided aortic arch; double outlet right ventricle; endocardial cushion defect;

> **Craniofacial:** microcephaly; bimaxillary protrusion; cleft lip; cleft palate; micrognathia; Robin sequence; flat philtrum; short nose; short palpebral fissures; epicanthal folds;

> **Immune:** DiGeorge sequence; immune deficiency;

> **Ocular:** small eyes; small optic disks;

> **Genitourinary:** labial hypoplasia; hypospadias; cryptorchidism; anomalous kidneys;

> **Integument:** hirsutism, especially on the back; hemangiomas;

> **Musculoskeletal:** scoliosis; bifid xiphoid; pectus excavatum or carinatum;

> **Limbs:** hypoplastic nails; characteristic palmar crease; radioulnar fusion; limited joint flexion; polydactyly; small hands and feet.

Natural History: Babies with fetal alcohol syndrome are typically small at birth. Growth then follows a steady, but below normal course. Babies with fetal alcohol syndrome are often irritable and may also be difficult to feed. Developmental milestones are all generally delayed, including speech and language. Chronic upper and lower respiratory infections are common. The infantile irritability does not persist into childhood in most cases.

Treatment Prognosis: The prognosis is dependent on the severity of cognitive impairment and brain malformation. In milder cases, the prognosis is excellent.

Differential Diagnosis: The heart, palatal, immune, and learning disorders in fetal alcohol syndrome are very similar to those found in **velo-cardio-facial syndrome.** Fetal hydantoin syndrome also shares many of the developmental, limb, and cardiac findings.

FG Syndrome

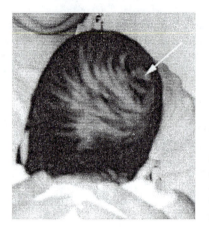

FG syndrome: Abnormal head shape with upsweeping hair and abnormal location of the hair whorl in an infant with FG syndrome.

Also Known As: Opitz-Kaveggia syndrome.

FG syndrome is an X-linked syndrome of mental retardation with speech, language, and hearing impairment as clinical features. The syndrome is rare, but is probably under-reported.

Major System(s) Affected: Central nervous system; growth; craniofacial; gastrointestinal; limbs; cardiac; integument; ocular; genital.

Etiology: X-linked inheritance. The gene has been mapped to Xq12-q21.31, but not identified.

Quick Clues: The ears have a simple architecture and the scalp hair is upsweeping.

Hearing Disorders: Sensorineural hearing loss occurs in approximately a third of cases.

Speech Disorders: A small number of patients with FG syndrome have severe retardation and do not develop speech, but most are moderately or mildly retarded and develop a characteristic pattern of talkativeness that is probably related to their overall temperament. Patients with FG syndrome are often overly affectionate and friendly much of the time, but then may erupt into temper tantrums and impulsive, disinhibited behavior with occasionally violent outbursts. Their speech may represent a part of their temperament disorder that includes flights of ideas resulting in long strings of emotional speech. Cleft palate is an uncommon finding in the syndrome, but may cause compensatory articulation patterns when present.

Feeding Disorders: Early feeding is often impaired by hypotonia. Airway obstruction or pulmonary disease may complicate early failure-to-thrive.

Voice Disorders: Wet hoarseness secondary to lower airway congestion is possible.

Resonance Disorders: Although hypernasality may occur in individuals with clefts, hyponasality is more common. Upper airway obstruction from lymphoid tissue hypertrophy is common and may result in hyponasality. Chronic mouth-open posture and vertical maxillary excess develop from a combination of nasal obstruction and facial hypotonia.

Language Disorders: Language is essentially always delayed commensurate with cognitive impairment.

Other Clinical Features:

Central nervous system: mental retardation; ADD and ADHD; absence or hypoplasia of the corpus callosum; cavum septum pellucidum; hypotonia; occasional seizures;

Growth: small stature in some cases;

Craniofacial: macrocephaly; plagiocephaly; delayed closure of the anterior fontanel; upsweeping scalp hair; hypertelorism; occasional cleft palate; vertical maxillary excess; protruding ears; overfolded helices;

Gastrointestinal: chronic constipation; imperforate or stenotic anus; megacolon;

Limbs: hypertrophic toe pads; broad thumbs and halluces;

Cardiac: ventriculoseptal defect; conotruncal heart anomalies;

Integument: depigmented and hyperpigmented areas

of skin arranged in linear streaks;

Ocular: exotropia; enlarged cornea;

Genitals: hypospadias; cryptorchidism.

Natural History: The anomalies are all static and present at birth. Development is globally slower than normal. Language will often develop in a burst of activity in early childhood.

Treatment Prognosis: Prognosis for communicative impairment is typically good. Behavior disorders, however, tend to get progressively worse with age.

Differential Diagnosis: Many of the anomalies in FG syndrome are similar to those seen in **velo-cardio-facial syndrome,** including the heart anomalies, behavior patterns, constipation, and genital anomalies. However, the pattern of inheritance in FG syndrome is clearly X-linked, unlike the autosomal dominant mode of inheritance in **velo-cardio-facial syndrome.**

Frontometaphyseal Dysplasia

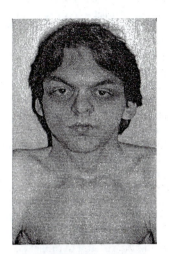
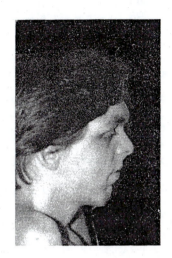

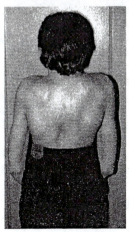

Frontometaphyseal dysplasia: Note prominent supraorbital ridge and kyphoscoliosis (bottom).

Also Known As:

Frontometaphyseal dysplasia is a rare syndrome of craniofacial skeletal overgrowth associated with generalized skeletal dysplasia.

Major System(s) Affected:
Craniofacial; skeletal; dental; respiratory; genitourinary.

Etiology: X-linked recessive inheritance. The gene has not been mapped or identified.

Quick Clues: The craniotubular skeletal dysplasias share some phenotypic characteristics, especially of the craniofacial complex. Because each is very rare, the recognition of the facial characteristics would lead to a differential diagnosis for these dysplasias. Frontometaphyseal dysplasia has a particularly prominent supraorbital ridge and with progression of the disorder, severe kyphoscoliosis.

Hearing Disorders: Mixed hearing loss is a consistent finding resulting from the combination of skeletal overgrowth and mastoid bone anomalies.

Speech Disorders: Speech production is impaired in both articulation and duration. The secondary teeth are typically congenitally missing, resulting in over-retained primary teeth and spacing problems that result in anterior distortions. Breath support is weak, resulting in weak acoustic production and shortened phrase length.

Feeding Disorders: Feeding is typically normal in infancy, but with age, airway compromise becomes more severe, resulting in difficulties with large, difficult to chew pieces of food. Subsequent dental abnormalities (absence of permanent dentition) may impair the ability to chew certain foods, thus prolonging the amount of time it takes to eat.

Voice Disorders: Hoarseness and breathiness are common.

Resonance Disorders: Resonance may be normal, or occasionally hyponasal secondary to nasal obstruction.

Language Disorders: Language and cognition are typically normal.

Other Clinical Features:

> **Craniofacial:** prominence of the forehead and supraorbital ridge; short lower third

face height with a prominent chin; multiple skeletal hyperostoses; sclerosis of the cranial bones;

Skeletal: metaphyseal dysplasia; kyphoscoliosis; progressive joint limitation and contractions; pectus carinatum;

Dental: congenitally missing permanent dentition; over-retained primary teeth;

Respiratory: pulmonary restriction; tracheal stenosis; subglottic stenosis; obstructive sleep apnea;

Genitourinary: cryptorchidism; hydronephrosis.

Natural History: Pulmonary restriction and subsequent poor breath support are progressive and related to severe deformity of the spine and ribs from progressive skeletal dysplasia. Hearing loss is

progressive. Chronic middle ear disease may also occur. Tracheal and subglottic stenoses begin in the second decade of life and become progressively worse. Obstructive sleep apnea also may begin in the second decade of life and is related to both craniofacial anomalies and lower airway anomalies.

Treatment Prognosis: Symptomatic treatment and palliative treatment can be beneficial because the progression of the disorder is not as rapid as in some other bony overgrowth syndromes. Of primary importance is good airway support. Therefore, efforts to limit the kyphoscoliosis should be made.

Differential Diagnosis: Craniometaphyseal dysplasia is similar, but the extracranial skeletal findings involve more metaphyseal flaring. In frontometaphyseal dysplasia, the prominence of the supraorbital ridge is a striking and distinctive feature.

Gernet Syndrome

Also Known As: Deafness-optic atrophy syndrome.

This is a relatively rare syndrome of progressive visual impairment and sensorineural hearing loss. Because there are a number of more common syndromes with the combination of visual impairment and sensorineural hearing deficits, it is likely that some individuals with Gernet syndrome are misdiagnosed.

Major System(s) Affected: Ocular; auditory.

Etiology: Autosomal dominant inheritance. The gene has not been mapped or identified.

Quick Clues: The association of progressive visual impairment is common with deafness. Gernet syndrome differs from the subtypes of Usher syndrome in that the visual impairment is not related to retinitis pigmentosa.

Hearing Disorders: Congenital severe to profound sensorineural hearing loss is the rule, but later onset and less severe hearing loss has also been documented in some af-

fected individuals. The hearing loss is stable. Vestibular function is normal.

Speech Disorders: Speech is impaired only by the accompanying hearing loss.

Feeding Disorders: Feeding is normal.

Voice Disorders: Voice is normal.

Resonance Disorders: Resonance is impaired only by the associated hearing loss.

Language Disorders: Language impairment may be associated with the severe to profound sensorineural hearing loss. In cases with later onset, language development has been normal.

Other Clinical Features:

> **Ocular:** progressive optic atrophy

Natural History: Optic atrophy varies at age of onset from childhood to the third decade of life. Hearing loss, although most often congenital, may have a later onset in childhood in milder expressions of the syndrome.

Treatment Prognosis: The most severe end of the spectrum of visual impairment occurs late in life and, until then, vision is typically adequate at least into middle age. Hearing loss is nonprogressive and may be amenable to amplification.

Differential Diagnosis: Optic atrophy occurs in a number of rare syndromes and may also be an isolated genetic trait. The association of visual impairment and hearing loss is found in the **Usher syndromes, Refsum syndrome,** and several other relatively common syndromes of hearing loss.

G

Gorlin-Chaudhry-Moss Syndrome

Also Known As:

Major System(s) Affected: Craniofacial; integument; dental; musculoskeletal; growth; genitourinary; central nervous system.

Etiology: Autosomal recessive inheritance. The gene has not been mapped or identified.

Quick Clues: A midline dimple in the chin and a low anterior hairline with coarse, thick, and abundant scalp hair are common and easily noticed.

Hearing Disorders: Conductive hearing loss is common.

Speech Disorders: Speech onset is delayed secondary to mild mental retardation.

Feeding Disorders: Feeding disorders have not been observed or documented.

Voice Disorders: Voice disorders have not been reported.

Resonance Disorders: Mild hyponasality may occur.

Language Disorders: Language is impaired.

Other Clinical Features:

Craniofacial: craniosynostosis; dimple in the midline of the chin; maxillary hypoplasia; downslanting eyes;

Integument: low anterior hairline; coarse hair; abundant scalp hair; hypertrichosis of the arms, legs, and back;

Dental: hypodontia; small teeth;

Musculoskeletal: short distal phalanges of all digits on the hands and feet; short metacarpals;

Growth: short stature;

Genitourinary: hypoplastic labia majora;

Central nervous system: cognitive impairment.

Natural History: The disorder is evident at birth. The facial features become more evident with time, but there is no substantial progression of the clinical features.

Treatment Prognosis: Early craniectomy may be necessary, but cognitive impairment exists independent of relieving increased intracranial pressure.

Differential Diagnosis: Crouzon syndrome exhibits craniosynostosis and maxillary deficiency, but does not have the integument findings or the cognitive impairment associated with Gorlin-Chaudhry-Moss syndrome.

G

Hajdu-Cheney Syndrome

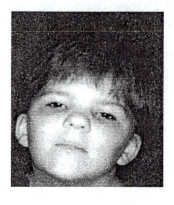

Hajdu-Cheney syndrome: Round, compressed facial appearance with short nose and anteverted nostrils.

Also Known As: Arthrodento-osteodysplasia.

Hajdu-Cheney syndrome is a rare disorder that probably represents a connective tissue dysplasia. The primary effects are skeletal and several of the anomalies have a direct impact on speech production. Recognition of the syndrome is critical because of progressive compression at the base of the skull that can cause hydrocephalus, and Arnold-Chiari anomaly that may result in death if untreated.

Major System(s) Affected: Skeletal; craniofacial; growth; dental; limbs; central nervous system; ocular.

Etiology: Autosomal dominant inheritance. The gene has not been mapped or identified.

Quick Clues: The craniofacial appearance of Hajdu-Cheney syndrome is distinctive, especially in relation to the shape of the cranium. The head appears disproportionately large with an especially prominent occiput. The face is vertically short.

Hearing Disorders: Both conductive and sensorineural hearing losses have been noted. Sensorineural loss is typically mild to moderate in severity.

Speech Disorders: Speech is typically impaired by a number of structural anomalies, including jaw and dental abnormalities. The dentition is lost early because of alveolar bone resorption and root exposure. The mandible undergoes progressive shortening of the ramus and condyle, resulting in shortening of the lower third of the face and micrognathia. Obligatory articulation disorders result from the lack of dentition and severe maxillary overjet. Lingual protrusion is typical. If skull base compression occurs and is not corrected surgically, there may be VIIth nerve compression and facial paresis.

Feeding Disorders: Early feeding is normal. Feeding in adolescence and adult life can be impaired by lack of dentition and shortening of the ramus and condyle of the mandible. The airway may become marginal and result in choking on large or chewy pieces of food. With progression of basilar compression, there may be a loss of sensation in the pharynx and larynx increasing the potential for aspiration.

Voice Disorders: Low, hoarse voice is a common finding, and breathiness may be present if cranial base compression occurs resulting in vocal cord paresis.

Resonance Disorders: Resonance begins normally, but if skull base compression occurs, hypernasality may result from nerve compression.

Language Disorders: Language development is normal.

Other Clinical Features:

Skeletal: osteoporosis; acroosteolysis; multiple bone fractures; wormian bones; kyphoscoliosis; vertebral anomalies;

Craniofacial: shortening of the mandibular ramus and blunting of the condyles with resorption of condylar bone; micrognathia; widely patent cranial sutures; occasional cleft palate; basilar impression causing impulsion of the cerebellum through the foramen magnum; protuberant ears; epicanthal folds; short nose and resulting long philtrum; low anterior hairline;

Growth: short stature;

Dental: loss of dentition and alveolar bone;

Limbs: dislocation of the patellas; joint laxity;

Central nervous system: potential for hydrocephalus;

potential for Arnold-Chiari anomaly;

Ocular: myopia; potential for optic atrophy; potential for nystagmus.

Natural History: The anomalies are present at birth, but the skeletal anomalies are progressive. Abnormalities of the skull base begin later in childhood and can become life threatening. Dental loss occurs in adolescence and is progressive as the alveolar bone is resorbed.

Treatment Prognosis: Intellect is normal and, with aggressive management, including early detection and surgical management of the basilar compression, the outcome can be good.

Differential Diagnosis: Pycnodysostosis has similar skeletal findings, including bone resorption, fractures and shortening of the ramus, and dental loss. However, the voice in pycnodysostosis is high pitched.

Harboyan Syndrome

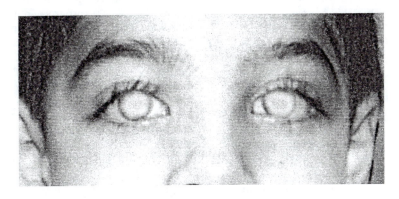

Harboyan syndrome: Opacified corneas in Harboyan syndrome.

Also Known As: Corneal dystrophy and perceptive deafness.

Opacifications of the cornea resulting in decreased vision are congenital in Harboyan syndrome. Hearing loss is of relatively late onset in most cases and is not accompanied by vestibular dysfunction.

Major System(s) Affected: Ocular; auditory.

Etiology: Autosomal recessive inheritance. The gene has not been mapped or characterized.

Quick Clues: The corneal opacities in Harboyan syndrome are visible to the naked eye. Therefore, the association of reduced vision caused by corneal clouding with sensorineural hearing loss should lead to the suspicion of Harboyan syndrome.

Hearing Disorders: Progressive bilateral sensorineural hearing loss is the rule, usually with onset in the second decade of life. Progression is relatively slow.

Speech Disorders: Speech is not typically impaired because of the late onset of the hearing impairment.

Feeding Disorders: Feeding disorders do not accompany Harboyan syndrome.

Voice Disorders: Voice disorders are not associated with Harboyan syndrome.

Resonance Disorders: Resonance is normal.

Language Disorders: Language is unaffected.

Other Clinical Features:

> **Ocular:** Congenital corneal opacification; edema of the stroma; slowly progressive loss of vision.

Natural History: Both the visual and hearing impairment are slowly progressive. The hearing loss is not typically detected until 10 years of age or later and the progression is slow.

Treatment Prognosis: The hearing loss is typically moderate to severe and is amenable to amplification. Because the progression is slow, the overall prognosis for hearing is good. Visual impairment also progresses slowly, but is present at birth, so that reduced acuity is always present. Surgical management later in life is possible should the progression be severe enough to cause marked impairment.

Differential Diagnosis: There are several genetic forms of corneal dystrophy that present as isolated anomalies. Because the hearing loss has a later onset, the diagnosis of Harboyan syndrome may be delayed until the hearing loss is detected. Corneal clouding also occurs in the lysosomal storage diseases, but in these syndromes, there are many other findings associated with the metabolic disorder.

Herrmann Syndrome

Also Known As: Photomyoclonus, diabetes mellitus, deafness, nephropathy, and cerebral dysfunction.

Herrmann syndrome is a rare disorder of hearing loss, neurologic disorders that contribute to speech and language impairment, and endocrine disease. The hearing loss is apparently caused by cochlear degeneration. This condition should not be confused with another disorder labeled as Herrmann syndrome that involves craniofacial and limb anomalies.

Major System(s) Affected: Endocrine; auditory; central nervous system; renal.

Etiology: The syndrome has been described as an autosomal dominant disorder because of vertical transmission on pedigree analysis. However, all cases have been inherited maternally and the symptoms are similar in some respects to other mitochondrial disorders. This may therefore represent a mitochondrial disorder. The pattern of inheritance could also be consistent with an X-linked dominant disorder, but there is no lethality in males.

Quick Clues: There are really no distinguishing physical characteristics in Herrmann syndrome. Therefore, the clinician needs to be attentive to medical history in order to draw the association between the specific form of seizures, diabetes mellitus, and the progressive degeneration associated with Herrmann syndrome.

Hearing Disorders: Progressive sensorineural hearing loss of variable severity has been linked to progressive cochlear degeneration. Onset of hearing loss may not be detected until the third or fourth decade of life.

Speech Disorders: Speech is dysarthric, sluggish, and articulation slurred.

Feeding Disorders: Feeding is not impaired.

Voice Disorders: Voice is normal.

119

Resonance Disorders: Resonance is mixed hyper/hyponasal of the type often seen in individuals with dysarthria.

Language Disorders: The onset of language is typically normal, but with age, there may be deterioration of function in association with seizures, dementia, and ataxia.

Other Clinical Features:

Endocrine: diabetes mellitus;

Auditory: progressive sensorineural hearing loss;

Central nervous system: photomyoclonic seizures; focal motor seizures; ataxia; nystagmus; dementia; depression;

Renal: nephropathy.

Natural History: The development and progression of Herrmann syndrome is highly variable. In some cases, the onset is very late and the progression is slow so that the overall effect is mild. In other cases, the onset is earlier and the progression more rapid with the disorder resulting in early demise.

Treatment Prognosis: In milder cases, palliative treatment is sufficient. In more severe cases, the progression of the disorder is inevitable and treatment is likely to have short term benefit.

Differential Diagnosis: Refsum syndrome has the association of progressive neurologic impairment and sensorineural deafness, but also has progressive skin anomalies and visual impairment. There are other mitochondrial disorders with similar presentations, including MERRF syndrome (Mitochondrial encephalopathy, myoclonus Epilepsy, Ragged-Red Fibers, and sensorineural hearing loss.

HMC Syndrome

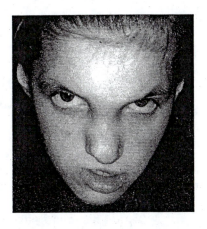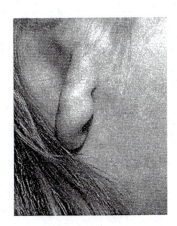

HMC syndrome: Note cleft and facial asymmetry associated with HMC syndrome (left) with microtia (right).

Also Known As: *Hypertelorism, Microtia, Clefting syndrome; Bixler syndrome.*

HMC syndrome is a rare, but probably under-reported syndrome that features craniofacial anomalies, conductive hearing loss, and renal anomalies. The syndrome may not be diagnosed frequently because many of its features overlap other easily recognized syndromes that are commonly seen in busy craniofacial centers.

Major System(s) Affected: Craniofacial; renal; musculoskeletal; cardiac; central nervous system.

Etiology: Autosomal recessive inheritance. The gene has not been mapped or identified.

Quick Clues: There is significant overlap of the physical findings in HMC syndrome with **oculo-auriculo-vertebral dysplasia.** Because essentially all individuals with HMC syndrome have cognitive impairment, but only a small percentage of patients with **oculo-auriculo-vertebral dysplasia** are mentally retarded, the presence of marked intellectual deficiency would include HMC as part of the differential diagnosis.

Hearing Disorders: Conductive hearing loss, maximal in ears with grade III microtia.

Speech Disorders: Speech onset may be delayed. Malocclusion occurs in essentially all cases including lateral open-bite, resulting in obligatory distortions or substitutions.

Feeding Disorders: Feeding disorders have not been reported, but cleft lip and palate may complicate early feeding attempts.

Voice Disorders: Voice has not been reported or observed to be abnormal.

Resonance Disorders: Resonance is hypernasal in cases with clefts that develop velopharyngeal insufficiency.

Language Disorders: Language impairment is commensurate with the degree of cognitive impairment.

Other Clinical Features:

> **Craniofacial:** hypertelorism; microtia; cleft lip and palate; facial asymmetry; micrognathia; microstomia; broad or bifid nasal tip; microcephaly;

> **Renal:** ectopic kidney; ureter stenosis;

> **Musculoskeletal:** vertebral anomalies; hypoplasia of the thenar muscle;

> **Cardiac:** ASD;

> **Central nervous system:** cognitive impairment.

Natural History: The anomalies are present at birth. Facial asymmetry may become more pronounced with age because the more severely affected side of the face will grow more slowly than the normal side.

Treatment Prognosis: Surgical management can resolve the craniofacial anomalies and, together with speech therapy, can result in resolution of speech impairment. Language correction is in large part dependent on the degree of cognitive impairment.

Differential Diagnosis: HMC syndrome has phenotypic overlap with two other syndromes often seen in craniofacial centers, including **oculo-auriculo-vertebral spectrum** (facial asymmetry, microtia, and clefting), and **craniofronto-nasal dysplasia syndrome** (hypertelorism, broad/bifid nose, cleft lip/palate).

Holoprosencephaly

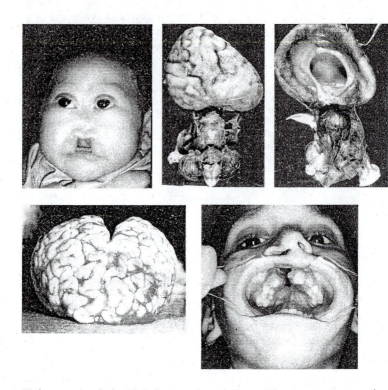

Holoprosencephaly: Facial expression of premaxillary agenesis type of holoprosencephaly and the associated brain anomalies (top row). At center is the brain of this baby who expired at five weeks of age. Note the lack of hemispheric differentiation and the presence of a single large central ventricle (right). The brain at the bottom left is an example of partially lobar holoprosencephaly with partial hemispheric differentiation. At bottom right is a milder expression with a single central incisor and near midline cleft of the primary palate.

Also Known As: DeMyer sequence; cyclopia; ethmocephaly; cebocephaly; arrhinencephaly; premaxillary agenesis; single central incisor syndrome; **Kallmann syndrome.**

Holoprosencephaly is a term used to describe a spectrum of disorders that involve primary brain anomalies of varying severity. In the most severe cases, there is a complete lack of septation of the brain resulting in a single holosphere without a normal ventricular system, known as alobar holoprosencephaly. In milder cases, there may be complete septation of the brain with partial absence or hypoplasia of some of the communicating tracts, and perhaps lack of development of the olfactory bulbs, known as lobar holoprosencephaly. Partial septation of the brain is known as partially lobar holoprosencephaly. The most severe forms are incompatible with life, but milder forms may have normal mentation and life span, but may exhibit growth deficiency (related to pituitary hypoplasia) or absence of the sense of smell.

Major System(s) Affected: Craniofacial; central nervous system; genitals; growth; endocrine; ocular.

Etiology: There are multiple etiologies for holoprosencephaly. A number of genes have been identified that result in this disorder, including deletions at 2p21, 7q36, 18p11, and 21q22.3. A number of single gene syndromes give rise to holoprosencephaly as a secondary sequence, including Meckel syndrome, **velo-cardio-facial syndrome,** and **Kallmann syndrome** among others. Chromosomal disorders may also result in holoprosencephaly as part of their symptom complexes, including trisomy 13, trisomy 18, and triploidy. Interstitial and terminal deletions have also resulted in holoprosencephaly, including deletions of 18p, 13q, and 2p.

Quick Clues: Severe cases of holoprosencephaly are obvious because of severe facial anomalies and brain malformations. It is unlikely that such cases will be seen for clinical assessments of hearing as many die in the early days or weeks of life. In milder forms, the eyes and teeth may provide valuable diagnostic clues, including coloboma of the iris, hypotelorism, and single central incisor.

Hearing Disorders: Hearing is likely to be impaired on a central basis in more severe cases, but measurement of hearing is difficult to assess reliably either behaviorally or electrophysiologically because of the severe brain anomalies. Holoprosencephaly often occurs in association with other craniofacial anomalies, including microtia, middle ear malformations, and cranial nerve anomalies, resulting in both sensorineural and conductive hearing loss.

Speech Disorders: Patients with lobar holoprosencephaly do not develop speech. Patients with partially lobar holoprosencephaly are unlikely to develop any expressive language. Individuals with lobar holoprosencephaly may develop speech, and may even have normal intellect. In those individuals who do develop speech, many are likely to have malocclusions, maxillary hypoplasia, class III malocclusions, and missing teeth leading to obligatory articulation errors.

Feeding Disorders: Feeding is severely impaired in cases with more severe brain anomalies. Failure-to-thrive is the rule based on severe neurologic abnormalities, including hypertonicity and spasticity with severe irritability.

Voice Disorders: Voice is normal in cases with verbal communication.

Resonance Disorders: Resonance may be hypernasal secondary to cleft palate (including submucous) or cleft lip and palate, both of which are common in the holoprosencephalic spectrum. Hyponasality may also occur related to a smaller than normal nasal cavity in some cases.

Language Disorders: Language development is absent in cases with severe brain anomalies. In less severe anomalies, language may still be absent, but is certainly severely impaired. In milder cases of lobar holoprosencephaly, language development may, on occasion, be normal.

Other Clinical Features:

Craniofacial: severe hypotelorism; cyclopia; single nostrils; absent midline facial structures; absent premaxilla with true median cleft lip; abnormal proboscis in place of nose; microcephaly; upslanting palpebral fissures;

Central nervous system: total or incomplete septation of the brain; absent olfactory tracts; absent corpus callosum and other communicating tracts; pituitary deficiency; lack of ability to maintain stasis; seizures; hypertonicity; hyperreflexia;

Genitals: hypogonadism;

Growth: short stature;

Endocrine: growth hormone deficiency; diabetes insipidus;

Ocular: iris, retinal, and optic nerve colobomas;

Other: many other somatic or craniofacial anomalies may be associated with holoprosencephaly because of the many potential causes and associated malformations with other syndromes.

Natural History: When the brain anomalies are severe, as in alobar holoprosencephaly, the prognosis for survival past the neonatal period is poor. Babies develop central apnea, have difficulty with temperature regulation, and usually expire within days or weeks. Cases that survive the neonatal period may live into adult years but be severely retarded and in a perpetual cachectic and spastic state. In milder cases, there may be global developmental delay, often severe. Some individuals have normal intellect and their prognosis is excellent.

Treatment Prognosis: Ranges from extremely poor to excellent, depending on the severity of the brain anomaly.

Differential Diagnosis: Binder syndrome has the appearance of hypotelorism and severe midface deficiency that resemble some forms of holoprosencephaly. Midline pseudocleft of the lip is seen in **oral-facial-digital syndrome.** However, holoprosencephaly has distinctive brain characteristics that can be detected with brain ultrasound, MR scan, or CT scan.

Hunter Syndrome

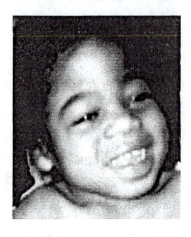

Hunter syndrome: Coarsening of the face in a child with the milder form (type B) of Hunter syndrome.

Also Known As: Mucopolysaccharidosis (MPS) type II; iduronate 2-sulfatase deficiency.

Hunter syndrome is the only mucopolysaccharidosis syndrome (or lysosomal storage disease) that is X-linked in etiology. A number of different mutations in the same gene have been discovered, and there are two subtypes of Hunter syndrome differentiated by severity. These two forms have been designated as MPS IIA (severe form) and MPS IIB (mild form). Life expectancy is significantly shortened in MPS IIA, but people with MPS IIB may live into the sixth or seventh decades of life. The features of Hunter syndrome are similar to those of the other mucopolysaccharidosis syndromes, including the postnatal onset of coarsening of the face, swelling of the joints, cognitive deficiency and deterioration, and respiratory difficulties. For a more detailed explanation of lysosomal storage diseases, see the entry for **Hurler syndrome.**

Major System(s) Affected: Growth; central nervous system; craniofacial; ocular; musculoskeletal; cardiopulmonary; integument; gastrointestinal.

Etiology: X-linked recessive inheritance. The gene has been mapped to Xq28 and has been labelled *IDS* (iduronate 2-sulfatase).

Quick Clues: The association of chronic respiratory illness with gradual coarsening of the facial features and progressive hearing loss are strong signals that an individual has Hunter syndrome or another of the lysosomal storage diseases. Hunter syndrome is distinct from other mucoploysaccharidoses in that it is X-linked, whereas the other forms are typically autosomal recessive so that only male children will be affected.

Hearing Disorders: As chronic congestion becomes more severe, conductive hearing loss occurs frequently with chronic middle ear effusion, complicated by thickened secretions and "glue ear." The frequency of middle ear effusion increases with age to the point where the problem is essentially continuous as the disease progresses. Hearing loss is progressive in both forms of the disorder.

Speech Disorders: In severe forms, early onset of speech milestones is normal, but with the onset of the clinical features, there is an initial arrest of development, and

subsequent degradation. Articulation becomes sluggish because the tongue becomes enlarged and the palate and alveolar ridges thickened, preventing normal tongue placement and movement. There is also neurologic degradation that contributes to dysarthria.

Feeding Disorders: Early feeding is normal. In childhood, children with the severe form begin to develop both respiratory compromise and anatomic alteration of the oral cavity making a normal diet difficult to tolerate. A change to a soft food diet may eventually be necessary and in the end-stage of the severe disorder, oral feeding may become impossible.

Voice Disorders: With the progression of the upper and lower airway congestion, there is a chronic wet hoarse voice.

Resonance Disorders: Resonance is initially normal, but may become hyponasal with age and the progression of the disorder.

Language Disorders: Early language development is initially normal for all cases. In the severe form, language development ceases in childhood and eventually deteriorates in adolescent years. In the milder form, language may remain normal into adult life.

Other Clinical Features:

> **Growth:** short stature (more severe in MPS IIA);

> **Central nervous system:** initial normal development followed by cognitive deficiency, mental retardation being ultimately severe in MPS IIA, but intellect is mildly impaired or normal in MPS IIB; hydrocephalus (in MPS IIA); seizures (MPS IIA); hyperactivity (MPS IIA);

> **Craniofacial:** coarse facies; thick lips; alveolar ridge hypertrophy; thickening of the palate;

> **Ocular:** papilledema; abnormal retinal pigmentation (MPS IIA); retinal degeneration (MPS IIA); corneal opacities (MPS IIB);

> **Musculoskeletal:** short neck (MPS IIA); carpal tunnel syndrome (MPS IIB); kyphosis; progressive joint stiffness; pes cavum;

> **Cardiopulmonary:** congestive heart failure; right-sided heart enlargement; valve disorders (MPS IIA); myocardial thickening (MPS IIA); coronary artery disease (MPS IIA);

> **Integument:** hirsutism; nodules on the shoulders, chest, and arms (MPS IIA);

> **Gastrointestinal:** liver and/or spleen enlargement (MPS IIA); diarrhea (MPS IIA); inguinal and umbilical hernias (MPS IIA).

Natural History: In the more severe form (MPS IIA), the disease becomes noticeable in early childhood and progresses rapidly with the majority of patients failing to survive past the age of 18 years. Cognitive, speech, language, and hearing functions all deteriorate with age. In the milder form (MPS IIB), the onset is later and the progression slower. Patients survive into adult life with only mild cognitive impairments or with normal intellect and language.

Treatment Prognosis: No effective treatments have yet been found for the severe form. Palliative treatment is indicated in milder cases, including treatment of middle ear fluid and respiratory illness.

Differential Diagnosis: The facial appearance and progressive nature of the disorder is similar to other lysosomal storage diseases and metabolic disorders. There are definitive molecular tests that can confirm the diagnosis of Hunter syndrome.

Hurler Syndrome

Also Known As: Mucopolysaccharidosis type I; alpha-L-iduronidase deficiency.

The lysosomal storage diseases, or mucopolysaccharidoses, are a group of genetic disorders involving metabolic abnormalities. These disorders are caused by deficiencies of a number of enzymes (lysosomal enzymes) that have the function of breaking down mucopolysaccharides, also known as glycosaminoglycans (GAGs). Mucopolysaccharides, or GAGs, are large, complex sugar molecules that play a role in the formation of the body's connective tissues. In normal individuals, the GAGs are continuously broken down for elimination by the lysosomal enzymes. If they are not broken down because of lysosomal deficiency, the GAGs are stored in the body's tissues. Therefore, these disorders are progressive and in the more severe forms, early death is expected. Hurler syndrome is one of the severe forms of mucopolysaccharidosis with an early and rapid downhill course. The missing enzyme in Hurler syndrome is alpha-L-iduronidase. Hurler syndrome is individually rare, with a birth frequency of approximately 1:100,000, but as a group, the mucopolysaccharidoses occur in at least 1:25,000 births.

Major System(s) Affected: Growth; central nervous system; craniofacial; ocular; musculoskeletal; limbs; cardiopulmonary; integument; gastrointestinal.

Etiology: Autosomal recessive inheritance. The gene has been mapped to 4p16.3 and labeled *alpha-L-iduronidase*. A number of other lysosomal storage diseases are allelic to Hurler syndrome, meaning that they are caused by different mutations in the same *alpha-L-iduronidase* gene. Scheie syndrome and Hurler-Scheie syndrome are allelic forms of mucopolysaccharidosis type I.

Quick Clues: The association of chronic respiratory illness with gradual coarsening of the facial features and progressive hearing loss are strong signals that an individual has Hurler syndrome or another of the lysosomal storage diseases.

Hearing Disorders: Conductive hearing loss secondary to chronic middle ear fluid becomes constant as the metabolic disease becomes more pronounced. The fluid in the middle ear is very thick and persitent.

Speech Disorders: Early developmental stages of vocalization are normal, but the disease progresses rapidly in late infancy/early toddler years. Psychomotor development is often normal in the first half year of life, and then slows dramatically before one year of age. Speech milestones cease to progress and little speech develops. Most individuals with Hurler syndrome succumb in childhood, usually before 10 years of age. Limited sound production is hampered by thickened alveolar ridges, a thickened palate, and chronic upper and lower airway obstruction.

Feeding Disorders: Early feeding is typically normal, but with the onset of noticeable symptoms, upper airway obstruction and advancing pulmonary disease, results in feeding difficulty. However, patients with Hurler syndrome typically appear "pudgy" and "puffy" because of the intracellular storage of GAGs. They become very inactive and overall caloric intake need not be large to maintain weight. Short stature results in the weight being disproportionately high compared to length. In childhood, the combination of oral cavity distortion and respiratory compromise make a normal diet impossible, and a change to soft diet becomes necessary. In late stages of the disease, alternative feeding procedures often become necessary.

Voice Disorders: Wet hoarseness and chronic congestion are common beginning at about three to six months of age, and become progressively worse with age.

Resonance Disorders: Hyponasality secondary to chronic nasal obstruction and enlargement of lymphoid tissue is very common.

Language Disorders: Language development reaches a near standstill by one to two years of age. The cognitive impairment caused by the metabolic disorder continues to progress until early demise within the first decade of life.

Other Clinical Features:

Growth: short stature of postnatal onset;

Central nervous system: progressive cognitive impairment;

Craniofacial: coarse facial features; thick lips; thickened alveolar ridges; thickened palate; macrocephaly; tongue enlargement;

Ocular: corneal opacities;

Musculoskeletal: thickened, stiff joints; kyphosis; short neck; thoracolumbar gibbus; hip flexion abnormalities;

Limbs: brachydactyly;

Cardiopulmonary: coronary artery disease; valvular stenosis; right-sided heart enlargement; cor pulmonale; obstructive apnea; pulmonary edema;

Integument: hirsutism;

Gastrointestinal/Abdominal: constipation; enlarged liver; enlarged spleen; umbilical hernia; inguinal hernias.

Natural History: Onset of the disorder is usually first noticed before six months of age, with progressive coarsening of the face, a slowing of motor development, stiffness of the joints, irritability, and chronic congestion. After six months, development slows dramatically, and by two years, becomes stagnant. Later in childhood, there is regression.

Treatment Prognosis: Extremely poor.

Differential Diagnosis: Hurler syndrome is differentiated from other lysosomal storage diseases and metabolic disorders based on laboratory tests specifying the enzyme that is abnormal.

Jackson-Weiss Syndrome

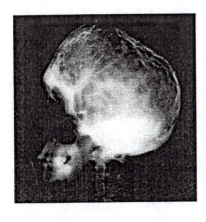

Jackson-Weiss syndrome: Craniosynostosis resulting in increased intracranial pressure and a "beaten copper" appearance of the skull bones in Jackson-Weiss syndrome.

Also Known As:

Jackson-Weiss syndrome is a syndrome of craniosynostosis that is more recently delineated than **Crouzon syndrome,** which it resembles. The syndrome is probably often misdiagnosed as **Crouzon** or **Pfeiffer syndrome.** Its true population prevalence is not known, but it probably occurs with lower frequency than **Crouzon syndrome.** Of interest, Jackson-Weiss is caused by a different mutation in the same gene responsible for **Crouzon syndrome.**

Major System(s) Affected:
Craniofacial; limbs.

Etiology: Autosomal dominant inheritance. The syndrome is caused by a mutation in the gene *FGFR2* (fibroblast growth factor receptor 2) that is located on chromosome 10q26.

Quick Clues: The facial manifestations in Jackson-Weiss syndrome are similar to those seen in **Crouzon syndrome.** The distinctive difference is the minor limb anomalies.

Hearing Disorders: Conductive hearing loss is an occasional finding.

Speech Disorders: Articulation is marked by obligatory anterior distortions related to Class III mal-occlusion and maxillary hypoplasia. The tongue is often forced to articulate in the mandibular arch because of constriction and hypoplasia of the maxilla.

Feeding Disorders: Early feeding may be impaired by nasal obstruction and airway compromise.

Voice Disorders: Voice is normal.

Resonance Disorders: Hyponasality is common secondary to nasal obstruction and a small nasopharyngeal cavity.

Language Disorders: Language development is typically normal.

Other Clinical Features:

> **Craniofacial:** craniosynostosis of multiple sutures; maxillary hypoplasia; mild exophthalmos;

> **Limbs:** broad halluces; soft tissue syndactyly of the second and third toes.

Natural History: At birth, some babies with Jackson-Weiss syndrome appear normal. With age, the maxillary hypoplasia becomes apparent and more pronounced as the mandible grows normally. The anterior fontanel may initially be open at birth even though craniosynostosis is already present in other sutures. The synostosis is not static, but slowly progressive. Therefore, presence of the anterior fontanel at birth should not be interpreted as meaning that the cranium is normal.

Treatment Prognosis: The prognosis is excellent. Cognitive impairment is not a clinical feature of Jackson-Weiss syndrome. The craniofacial anomalies can be managed surgically.

Differential Diagnosis: Craniosynostosis and maxillary hypoplasia are the key findings in **Crouzon syndrome,** but are more severe and exorbitism is common in **Crouzon,** whereas there is only mild bulging of the eyes in Jackson-Weiss syndrome. Soft tissue syndactyly is common in **Saethre-Chotzen syndrome,** but the craniosynostosis and facial anomalies are different from Jackson-Weiss. Broad halluces are common in **Pfeiffer syndrome,** but broad thumbs are not found in Jackson-Weiss, as they are in **Pfeiffer.**

Johanson-Blizzard Syndrome

Also Known As: Nasal alar hypoplasia, hypothyroidism, pancreatic achylia, and congenital deafness.

Johanson-Blizzard syndrome is rare but easily recognized because of the distinctive facial manifestations and endocrine disease. Female cases have predominated, but autosomal recessive inheritance has been confirmed by several pedigrees with unaffected parents and both male and female affected children.

Major System(s) Affected: Craniofacial; growth; central nervous system; endocrine; gastrointestinal; genitourinary; dental.

Etiology: Autosomal recessive inheritance. The gene has not been mapped or identified.

Quick Clues: The hypoplasia of the rims of the alar cartilages at the base of the nose is a distinctive and easily recognized anomaly associated with Johanson-Blizzard syndrome. The short stature and mental retardation also associated with the syndrome help to confirm the diagnosis.

Hearing Disorders: Severe or profound sensorineural hearing loss is the rule with Mondini type anomaly of the cochlea.

Speech Disorders: Speech production is severely limited in many, if not most, cases because of the combined effects of severe or profound sensorineural hearing loss and cognitive impairment. In some cases, there is very limited speech production, especially in the small sample of cases with normal intellect. However, in these cases, "deaf speech" is the norm.

Feeding Disorders: Although feeding is not impaired per se, weight gain is slow because of malabsorption and is often labeled as "failure-to-thrive." Severe cognitive impairment may also result in hypotonia in infancy. After the age of dental eruption, the teeth are anomalous or absent and chewing certain foods may be very difficult.

Voice Disorders: Voice disorders have not been observed or reported.

Resonance Disorders: Resonance is disordered secondary to "deaf speech" in those who have some speech, but in general, there may be a cul-de-sac quality to speech because of a constricted anterior nasal cavity from alar hypoplasia.

Language Disorders: Language is often severely impaired secondary to cognitive deficiency. Many patients have IQ scores below 50.

Other Clinical Features:

> **Craniofacial:** hypoplasia of the nasal alae; beak-like nose; delayed closure of the anterior fontanel; short anterior cranial base; maxillary hypoplasia;

> **Growth:** postnatal growth deficiency;

> **Central nervous system:** cognitive deficiency, often severe; abnormal gyri in the the cerebral cortex; neuronal disorganization;

> **Endocrine:** hypothyroidism; pancreatic insufficiency with malabsorption;

> **Gastrointestinal:** imperforate or anteriorly displaced anus;

> **Genitourinary:** double uterus; bicornate uterus; enlarged clitoris; micropenis; cryptorchidism; rectovaginal fistula;

> **Dental:** absent or anomalous secondary dentition; abnormal primary dentition;

> **Integument:** scalp defects; hypoplastic nipples; coarse and sparse scalp hair.

Natural History: Early failure-to-thrive is essentially constant because of malabsorption. Coupled with severe cognitive impairment and hypotonia, many infants do not survive, and these effects last into childhood. The pancreatic and endocrine disorders are progressive and become persistent medical problems.

Treatment Prognosis: In many cases, the prognosis is extremely poor, especially those where the cognitive impairment is severe. Even in cases with normal mentation, the endocrine disorders may significantly impair the quality and quantity of life.

Differential Diagnosis: Malabsorption is a feature of a number of syndromes, including Schwachman syndrome, but none has the distinctive facial appearance associated with Johanson-Blizzard syndrome. Hypoplasia of the nasal alae is found in trichorhinophalangeal syndrome and oculodento-osseous syndrome, but these syndromes do not have the same endocrine disorders.

J

Johnson-McMillin Syndrome

Also Known As: Johnson neuroectodermal syndrome; alopecia-anosmia-deafness-hypogonadism syndrome.

Johnson-McMillin syndrome is a rare multiple anomaly disorder that has a great deal of phenotypic overlap with other more common syndromes. It is therefore possible that this disorder is under-reported and often diagnosed as another syndrome.

Major System(s) Affected: Craniofacial; central nervous system; growth; genital; cardiac; integument.

Etiology: Autosomal dominant inheritance. The gene has not been mapped or identified.

Quick Clues: The combination of alopecia, hypohidrosis, facial asymmetry, and external ear malformations is distinctive to Johnson-McMillin syndrome. Although a rare disorder, it is likely that some cases are misdiagnosed as **oculo-auriculo-vertebral dysplasia.**

Hearing Disorders: Conductive hearing loss secondary to external and middle ear malformations is common.

Speech Disorders: Speech onset is delayed in the cases that show cognitive impairment. Mild micrognathia may occasionally contribute to misarticulations. Cleft palate can result in compensatory articulation secondary to velopharyngeal insufficiency.

Feeding Disorders: Early feeding may be complicated by cleft palate and mild hypotonia in some cases. Otherwise, feeding is typically normal.

Voice Disorders: Voice may be hoarse secondary to hypohidrosis.

Resonance Disorders: Resonance may be hypernasal secondary to cleft palate and velopharyngeal insufficiency.

Language Disorders: Cognitive impairment is an occasional finding that contributes to a commensurate delay and disorder of language. Congenital conductive hearing loss caused by middle ear anomalies may also contribute.

Other Clinical Features:

Craniofacial: cleft palate; facial asymmetry; micrognathia; facial nerve paresis;

Central nervous system: anosmia; mild cognitive impairment;

Growth: mild short stature;

Genital: hypogonadism secondary to pituitary deficiency;

Cardiac: heart anomalies;

Integument: hypohidrosis; alopecia; café-au-lait spots on the trunk.

Natural History: The anomalies in the syndrome are static and present at birth. Growth deficiency is secondary to the primary hormone deficiency.

Treatment Prognosis: Good to excellent. Patients may be treated symptomatically for all the disorders expressed in the syndrome with good outcomes, including hormone deficiency.

Differential Diagnosis: The anomalies of the external and middle ear in association with asymmetric facies and facial nerve paresis is found in **oculo-auriculo-vertebral dysplasia (OAV),** as is cleft palate. However, the integumentary and genital anomalies are not a feature of **OAV.** Alopecia and hypohidrosis in association with cleft palate is common in AEC syndrome and Rapp-Hodgkin syndrome, but neither of these disorders are associated with anosmia or growth deficiency with hypogonadism.

Kallmann Syndrome

Also Known As: Hypogonadotropic hypogonadism and anosmia; anosmic hypogonadism; dysplasia olfactogenitalis of de Morsier.

Kallmann syndrome refers to a group of disorders with a number of different etiologies that result in the association of anosmia, hypogonadism, and cleft lip and palate. There are a series of allelic variants that are X-linked, and there are probably autosomal recessive and autosomal dominant forms, as well. The X-linked variety is most common with an estimated incidence of 1:10,000 males. The syndrome makes up a significant percentage of males with hypogonadism.

Major System(s) Affected: Central nervous system; endocrine; craniofacial; genital; growth.

Etiology: The majority of cases show X-linked recessive inheritance. The gene has been mapped to Xp22.3.

Quick Clues: Although it is not often asked in the process of obtaining a history, the presence of anosmia is a strong indication that Kallmann syndrome may be the correct diagnosis. Because hypotelorism is often associated with anosmia, information about the sense of smell should be obtained when the eyes are close-set, and when cleft lip and palate are present.

Hearing Disorders: Sensorineural, conductive, and mixed hearing loss have all been observed. The majority of cases of hearing loss have been mild bilateral sensorineural.

Speech Disorders: Speech is variable, ranging from normal to severely impaired, with neurological components, including marked dysarthria. In the majority of cases with clefts, there are obligatory misarticulations related to malocclusion, missing teeth, and maxillary hypoplasia. Compensatory articulation may also occur secondary to cleft palate and velopharyngeal insufficiency.

Feeding Disorders: Feeding may be impaired by the cleft anomalies, and there is occasional mild infantile hypotonia. Weight gain may be slow, based on pituitary factors.

Voice Disorders: Voice is typically high pitched.

Resonance Disorders: Resonance may be hypernasal secondary to clefting and velopharyngeal insufficiency.

Language Disorders: Language may be delayed or impaired in some cases, based on overall mild developmental delay.

Other Clinical Features:

> **Central nervous system:** anosmia; hypothalamic gonadotropic-releasing hormone deficiency; occasional ataxia; occasional cognitive deficiency;

> **Endocrine:** impaired FSH and LH secretion; hypogonadotropic hypogonadism; decreased expression of secondary sexual characteristics;

> **Craniofacial:** cleft lip and/ or palate; maxillary deficiency; Genital: micropenis; cryptorchidism; testicular atrophy;

> **Growth:** occasional mild short stature; gynecomastia.

Natural History: The hypogonadism becomes more noticeable with age, as does maxillary deficiency. All other anomalies are present at birth and static.

Treatment Prognosis: Once identified, the prognosis is good and all anomalies can be treated symptomatically.

Differential Diagnosis: Anosmia and hypogonadism are common in **Johnson-McMillin syndrome,** but Kallmann syndrome does not have alopecia as a common finding. Hypogonadism may also occur in milder forms of **holoprosencephaly.**

Kartagener Syndrome

Also Known As: Dextrocardia, bronchiectasis, and sinusitis; Siewert syndrome; ciliary dyskinesia; immotile cilia syndrome.

Kartegener syndrome is regarded as the triad of situs inversus, ciliary immotility, and bronchiectasis. Situs inversus, the transposition of the body's organs to the side opposite of normal, is a fairly common anomaly that has no practical effect on health. However, ciliary immotility does cause chronic respiratory complications that need careful attention.

Major System(s) Affected: Respiratory; internal organs; reproductive.

Etiology: Autosomal recessive inheritance. The gene has not been mapped or identified.

Quick Clues: A history of situs inversus and dextrocardia in association with chronic respiratory illness should raise the suspicion of Kartegener syndrome.

Hearing Disorders: Conductive hearing loss secondary to chronic middle ear effusions and "glue ear" are common throughout life because of the effects of ciliary dyskinesia and resulting upper and lower airway congestion.

Speech Disorders: Speech is essentially normal, but can be affected by chronic congestion causing some articulation to be overly "moist."

Feeding Disorders: Early feeding is usually normal unless there is a very early onset of the respiratory symptoms that cause nasal obstruction and respiratory difficulties. In cases of very early onset, feeding may be compromised by respiratory difficulty. In later life, chronic congestion and nasal obstruction by polyps or mucus can cause choking, lack of taste (because of secondary anosmia), and decrease of appetite.

Voice Disorders: Wet hoarseness is nearly constant.

Resonance Disorders: Hyponasality secondary to nasal obstruction is common.

144

Language Disorders: Language development is normal.

Other Clinical Features:

Respiratory: immotile cilia; chronic sinusitis; absent frontal sinuses; bronchiectasis; asthma;

Internal organs: situs inversus; dextrocardia;

Reproductive: male infertility related to immotile sperm.

Natural History: The onset of the respiratory symptoms is variable. Situs inversus is asymptomatic, but is usually detected on normal clinical examination because of abnormal location of heart sounds.

Treatment Prognosis: Typically, the long term prognosis is very good. With aggressive respiratory therapy (postural drainage, chest physiotherapy, and coughing), longevity is not typically affected. Aggressive use of antibiotics is also recommended for even trivial illnesses. In some severe cases, heart-lung transplant may be recommended.

Differential Diagnosis: Situs inversus occurs as an isolated anomaly with no respiratory disorders. Dextrocardia is associated with a number of malformation syndromes when not accompanied by transposition of the other organs.

K

Kearns-Sayre Syndrome

Also Known As: Oculocraniosomatic syndrome; ophthalmoplegia-plus syndrome; mitochondrial cytopathy; chronic progressive external ophthalmoplegia with myopathy.

Kearns-Sayre syndrome is one of a small handful of progressive mitochondrial diseases with neurologic degeneration. The communicative implications are significant in both the speech and hearing realms. Mitochondrial disorders are inherited only from the mother because the genes are located in the mitochondria which are cytoplasmic, not nuclear, structures. All the cytoplasm of a fertilized zygote is maternal because the sperm has essentially no cytoplasm, only the nuclear material carrying the paternal chromosome haplotype.

Major system(s) affected: Growth; ocular; central nervous system; peripheral nervous system; endocrine; cardiac.

Etiology: Mitochondrial genetic alteration, probably a deletion of mitochondrial DNA.

Quick Clues: At the onset, mitochondrial disorders do not show any physical findings that would be considered distinctive. The abnormal eye movements in Kearns-Sayre syndrome might be the only early signs visible.

Hearing Disorders: High frequency sensorineural hearing loss is one of the first signs of the onset of the disorder. The hearing loss is progressive, but the deterioration is slow.

Speech Disorders: Early development of speech is normal. As the neurologic symptoms progress, facial, pharyngeal, and laryngeal weaknesses are expressed. Myopathic weakness is progressive, resulting in weak oral contacts and sluggish articulation.

Feeding Disorders: After the onset of myopathy, dysphagia becomes progressive and eventually severe. Feeding becomes progressively more difficult because of poor oral coordination. Eventually, seizures and transient stroke-like episodes become frequent and interfere with feeding.

Voice Disorders: Voice becomes initially hoarse, and then eventually becomes progressively breathy and weak.

Resonance Disorders: With the onset of myopathy, hypernasality becomes evident and progressively more severe.

Language Disorders: Language is initially normal. With age and the progression of seizures, there are aphasia-like episodes with deterioration of language.

Other Clinical Features:

Growth: short stature;

Ocular: ophthalmoplegia; retinal pigmentary degeneration; ptosis; eventual complete oculomotor paralysis;

Central nervous system: ataxia; hyperactive reflexes; cognitive deficiency; eventual dementia;

Peripheral nervous system: myopathy; peripheral neuropathy; sensory loss;

Endocrine: delayed secondary sexual characteristics; elevated blood sugar;

Cardiac: conduction defects; cardiomyopathy.

Natural History: The age of onset is variable. In general, the earlier the onset, the more severe the progression. The process in unrelenting, although relatively slow. Cardiac conduction defects often result in early death.

Treatment Prognosis: The disorder can not be treated successfully in either a palliative or definitive manner.

Differential Diagnosis: There are a number of mitochondrial syndromes that have associated hearing loss, including Borud syndrome, Cutler syndrome, **Herrmann syndrome,** MERRF syndrome, and Treft syndrome. However, the ophthalmic symptoms associated with Kearns-Sayre syndrome distinguish it from other mitochondrial disorders.

Keutel Syndrome

Also Known As: Pulmonic stenosis, brachytelephalangism, and calcification of cartilages.

This is a very rare syndrome with voice and hearing disorders. Fewer than 20 cases have been documented. The effect on voice is related to calcification of the laryngeal cartilages that results in abnormal mobility and articulation of the laryngeal structures.

Major System(s) Affected: Craniofacial; respiratory; skeletal; cardiopulmonary; central nervous system.

Etiology: Autosomal recessive inheritance. The gene has not been mapped or idenitified.

Quick Clues: Blunting of the finger tips and a depressed nasal tip are obvious clues to this rare syndrome.

Hearing Disorders: Sensorineural hearing loss is common.

Speech Disorders: Obligatory anterior articulation distortions and substitutions are likely related to maxillary hypoplasia and Class III malocclusion.

Feeding Disorders: Early failure-to-thrive may occur secondary to pulmonic stenosis and decreased vitality. However, in most cases, feeding is normal.

Voice Disorders: Voice is hoarse related to calcification of the laryngeal cartilages.

Resonance Disorders: Resonance is normal.

Language Disorders: Language is impaired in some cases secondary to cognitive impairment.

Other Clinical Features:

> **Craniofacial:** maxillary hypoplasia; depressed nasal tip;

> **Respiratory:** calcification of the larynx; calcification of the trachea;

> **Skeletal:** short terminal phalanges of all digits; calcified rib cartilage;

Cardiopulmonary: pulmonic stenosis, heart anomalies;

Central nervous system: occasional cognitive impairment.

Natural History: So few cases have been reported that it is not possible to know the exact nature of the progression of the disorder. However, the calcification is probably mildly progressive.

Treatment Prognosis: Unknown.

Differential Diagnosis: Maxillary hypoplasia with a depressed nasal tip is common in Binder syndrome. However, patients with Binder syndrome do not have respiratory or cardiac anomalies. Anomalies of the trachea associated with maxillary hypoplasia and a short nose is seen in **Stickler syndrome,** but the cartilages in **Stickler syndrome** are too soft, rather than calcified.

Klein-Waardenburg Syndrome

Also Known As: Waardenburg, syndrome, type III.

Klein-Waardenburg syndrome expresses more extracranial anomalies than the other forms of Waardenburg syndrome. It is also the only form of the Waardenburg-labeled disorders that has cognitive impairment as a feature.

Major System(s) Affected: Integument; ocular; musculoskeletal; central nervous system; gastrointestinal; craniofacial.

Etiology: Contiguous gene syndrome with autosomal dominant inheritance mapped to 2q35.

Quick Clues: Limb contractures associated with white forelock, telecanthus, and cognitive impairment are indicative of Klein-Waardenburg syndrome.

Hearing Disorders: Sensorineural hearing loss.

Speech Disorders: Severe or profound hearing loss compounded by cognitive impairment may result in speech impairment or severely delayed speech development.

Feeding Disorders: Feeding impairment related to Hirschsprung aganglionic megacolon is common.

Voice Disorders: Voice disorders have not been reported or observed.

Resonance Disorders: Resonance disorders are not found unless caused by congenital deafness.

Language Disorders: Language may be affected by hearing loss and cognitive impairment.

Other Clinical Features:

> **Integument:** white forelock; hypopigmentation of the skin;
>
> **Ocular:** telecanthus (dystopia canthorum); blepharophimosis;
>
> **Musculoskeletal:** flexion contractures; carpal fusions; syndactyly; winged scapulae;
>
> **Central nervous system:** cognitive impairment; microcephaly; spastic paraplegia;

Gastrointestinal: Hirschsprung aganglionic megacolon;

Craniofacial: broad nasal root.

Natural History: The anomalies associated with Klein-Waardenburg syndrome are congenital and static. Cognitive impairment and spastic paraplegia are the most serious disorders, but are not progressive.

Treatment Prognosis: Amplification for hearing loss is recommended. The cognitive impairment is related to underdevelopment of the brain and structural anomaly.

Differential Diagnosis: White forelock, sensorineural hearing loss, and Hirschsprung aganglionic megacolon are associated with other forms of **Waardenburg syndrome,** but Klein-Waardenburg differs with respect to the presence of cognitive deficiency.

Kniest Syndrome

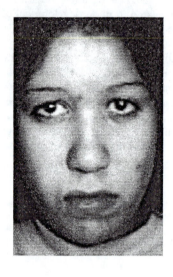

Kniest syndrome: Characteristic facial appearance.

Also Known As: Kniest dysplasia; metatropic dysplasia II; metatropic dwarfism, type II.

Kniest dysplasia is one of the syndromes of short stature that is frequently associated with cleft palate. Clefting is found in over half the patients with Kniest syndrome. A number of genetic mutations in the same gene causes this skeletal dysplasia. **Stickler syndrome** and **spondyloepiphyseal dysplasia congenita** are caused by different sets of mutations in the same gene (*COL2A1*).

Major System(s) Affected: Growth; craniofacial; ocular; skeletal.

Etiology: Autosomal dominant inheritance. The gene has been mapped to the long arm of chromosome 12 and has been identified as a collagen 2 gene, *COL2A1*.

Quick Clues: A depressed nasal root and round face are common minor facial anomalies in all the connective tissue dysplasias caused by *COL2A1* mutations (Kniest syndrome, **Stickler syndrome,** and **spondyloepiphyseal dysplasia congenita**).

Hearing Disorders: Approximately 15% to 25% of individuals with Kniest syndrome have sensorineural hearing loss, usually high frequency. Conductive hearing loss secondary to middle ear effusion is common in those cases with cleft palate.

Speech Disorders: Children with Kniest syndrome may develop compensatory articulation patterns secondary to cleft palate and velopharyngeal insufficiency.

Feeding Disorders: Early feeding may be impaired by upper airway obstruction caused by micrognathia and Robin sequence. Resolution of the airway problems resolves the feeding disorder.

Voice Disorders: Voice may be mildly hoarse related to lax connective tissue in the larynx.

Resonance Disorders: Resonance may be hypernasal secondary to cleft palate.

Language Disorders: Language development is typically normal.

Other Clinical Features:

> **Growth:** short stature;
>
> **Craniofacial:** macrocephaly; maxillary and mandibular hypoplasia; round facies; depressed nasal root; Robin sequence;
>
> **Ocular:** myopia; tendency toward retinal detachment; strabismus; cataracts;
>
> **Skeletal:** flattened vertebrae (platyspondyly); thin joint spaces; joint limitation; joint enlargement; club foot; lordosis; odontoid hypoplasia leading to the risk of atlanto-axial instability.

Natural History: The skeletal dysplasia and short stature become evident in infancy. Robin sequence is possible, but does not occur with as high a frequency as in other *COL2A1* disorders such as **Stickler syndrome** and **spondyloepiphyseal dysplasia congenita.** There is progressive deformation of the skeleton with age, including the potential for pulmonary restriction because of the spinal anomalies. Atlanto-axial instability may be present so that cervical spine radiographs need to be done and hyperextension of the neck avoided.

Treatment Prognosis: The skeletal dysplasia cannot be treated, but in general, the prognosis is good, including normal speech and language development.

Differential Diagnosis: Spondyloepiphyseal dysplasia congenita is another syndrome of short stature, Robin sequence, round facial appearance, and cleft palate. However, the radiographic findings are different and the type of X-ray findings are highly diagnostic of Kniest syndrome.

LADD Syndrome

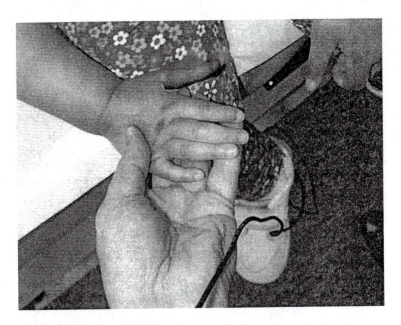

LADD syndrome: Abnormal digitalized thumb in LADD syndrome.

Also Known As: Levy-Hollister syndrome.

LADD is an acronym for Lacrimo-auriculo-dento-digital syndrome as a description of the major features of this relatively rare multiple anomaly disorder. The major features cited in the acronym are lacrimal duct anomalies, external ear malformation, hypoplastic teeth, and abnormal curvature of the fingers (clinodactyly) and thumb anomalies.

Major System(s) Affected: Craniofacial; ocular; musculoskeletal; dental; genitourinary.

Etiology: Autosomal dominant inheritance. The gene has not been mapped or identified.

Quick Clues: Thumb anomalies are striking with either partial duplication or long tapered triphalangeal thumbs.

Hearing Disorders: Hearing loss is variable and may be purely sensorineural, purely conductive, or mixed. Severity is also variable and cases with hearing loss have ranged from mild to severe impairment. Otosclerosis and/or ossicular anomalies are possible findings.

Speech Disorders: Speech production has been normal except in those cases where the severity of the hearing loss has been sufficient to impair articulation.

Feeding Disorders: Feeding disorders are not a feature of LADD syndrome.

Voice Disorders: Voice disorders are not a feature of LADD syndrome.

Resonance Disorders: Resonance may be impaired if hearing loss is severe.

Language Disorders: Language development has typically been normal except for those cases with the most severe hearing loss.

Other Clinical Features:

> **Craniofacial:** small cup-shaped auricles; asymmetric ears; absent or anomalous parotid and salivary glands;

> **Ocular:** lacrimal duct obstruction, hypoplasia, or aplasia; absent lacrimal puncta; dacryocystitis; recurrent conjunctivitis; absence of tearing;

> **Musculoskeletal:** duplication of the thumb tip; triphalangeal thumbs, tapered thumbs; long digitalized thumbs; short phalanges of all fingers; shortened radius; radioulnar synostosis; syndactyly; clinodactyly; broad halluces with occasional bifurcation;

> **Dental:** hypodontia of both the primary and secondary dentition; peg-shaped teeth; hypoplastic enamel; discolored teeth;

> **Genitourinary:** renal anomalies; hypospadias.

Natural History: The absence of tearing can lead to secondary eye problems, including chronic infection of the lacrimal system and conjunctiva. Because the teeth have thin enamel, severe and rapid decay is common with resulting loss of teeth and need for prosthetic replacement. Hearing loss is typically static unless there is progressive otosclerosis.

Treatment Prognosis: The prognosis is generally good. The eye problems can be treated both preventively and acutely without resulting harm to the globe. Dental anomalies can be treated prosthetically or with appropriate restorations. Surgical correction is possible for the limb anomalies and for lacrimal duct obstruction.

Differential Diagnosis: Limb findings with asymmetric or malformed ears is found in **Townes-Brocks syndrome,** but the range of other anomalies in **Townes-Brocks** is more severe, especially with regard to the craniofacial complex. Ear tags and pits are also present in **Townes-Brocks syndrome. BOR syndrome** has the association of hearing loss, external ear anomalies, and renal anomalies, but typically has the presence of preauricular pits.

Langer-Giedion Syndrome

Also Known As: Trichorhinophalangeal syndome, Type II.

Langer-Giedion is a well-recognized multiple anomaly syndrome that was initially grouped with another similar disorder, trichorhinophalangeal syndrome (now labeled trichorhinophalangeal syndrome type I), but was subsequently recognized to be a distinct and separate entity with some phenotypic overlap. It has since been found that Langer-Giedion syndrome is a contiguous gene disorder with the deletion from the long arm of chromosome 8 encompassing the single gene responsible for trichorhinophalangeal syndrome type I. Therefore, Langer-Giedion syndrome represents an expanded phenotype involving other genes surrounding the trichorhinophalangeal syndrome gene.

Major System(s) Affected: Skeletal; limbs; integument; craniofacial; central nervous system; genitourinary.

Etiology: Autosomal dominant inheritance. Langer-Giedion is caused by a contiguous gene deletion at 8q24.11-q24.13.

Quick Clues: A long pear-shaped nose with a bulbous tip is characteristic and when associated with digital anomalies (clinodactyly), the combination is distinctive.

Hearing Disorders: Sensorineural and mixed hearing loss occur in Langer-Giedion syndrome. The sensorineural component is progressive and may be moderate to severe.

Speech Disorders: Speech is typically delayed disproportionate to the degree of cognitive impairment. There are no specific articulation disorders characteristic of the syndrome.

Feeding Disorders: Feeding in infancy is nearly a constant problem and is related to the combined effects of retrognathia and hypotonia.

Voice Disorders: Voice is typically normal.

Resonance Disorders: Resonance is normal.

Language Disorders: Language is delayed, especially in terms of expressive language.

Other Clinical Features:

Skeletal: multiple exostoses; hyperextensible joints; cone-shaped epiphyses in the hands;

Limbs: clinodactyly of the fingers;

Integument: sparse scalp hair; thick eyebrows; redundant skin;

Craniofacial: bulbous nose; broad nasal root; prominent philtrum; microcephaly; micrognathia;

Central nervous system: cognitive impairment; hypotonia;

Genitourinary: G-U reflux; persistent cloaca;

Other: prune belly.

Natural History: The diagnosis may be difficult at birth because of the absence of hair in many newborns. The skeletal and facial features become more pronounced with age. Feeding difficulties are common in infancy, but are not syndrome specific, nor are they different problems from those found in other disorders with hypotonia and retrognathia.

Treatment Prognosis: Symptomatic treatment for the hearing and speech disorders are indicated and patients do respond to appropriate speech-language stimulation.

Differential Diagnosis: Trichorhinophalangeal syndrome type I shares many of the same phenotypic features as Langer-Giedion syndrome. The facial manifestations, hypotonia, and feeding difficulties in Langer-Giedion are similar to those found in **velo-cardio-facial syndrome,** but cleft palate is not a feature of Langer-Giedion.

Larsen Syndrome

Also Known As:

Larsen syndrome is a disorder of joint dislocations and cleft palate that has been reported to occur in two forms: autosomal recessive and autosomal dominant. The clinical presentation of the two forms are essentially the same, so they will be described as a single entry.

Major System(s) Affected: Musculoskeletal; craniofacial; limbs.

Etiology: The autosomal dominant form has been mapped to 3p21.1-014.1. The gene has been labeled *LAR1*. The autosomal recessive form has not been mapped. Though Larsen syndrome involves multiple joint dislocations, neither the dominant nor recessive forms has been linked to any of the collagen or fibrillin genes that have typically been associated with joint and skeletal abnormalities.

Quick Clues: Multiple and severe joint dislocations.

Hearing Disorders: Conductive hearing loss occurs secondary to dislocations of the ossicles. Abnormalities of the footplate of the stapes also occur. Mixed and sensorineural hearing loss have been observed infrequently.

Speech Disorders: Compensatory articulation patterns may occur secondary to cleft palate and velopharyngeal insufficiency.

Feeding Disorders: Early feeding may be complicated by clefting, but is otherwise normal.

Voice Disorders: Voice is normal.

Resonance Disorders: Hypernasal resonance is common secondary to cleft palate.

Language Disorders: Language and intellect are normal.

Other Clinical Features:

> **Musculoskeletal:** multiple congenital joint dislocations; scoliosis;

> **Craniofacial:** flattened midface; cleft palate;

Limbs: dislocation of the tibia; brachydactyly; extra carpal bones.

Natural History: The joint dislocations are present at birth and others may develop shortly after. Lax joints persist throughout life.

Treatment Prognosis: Surgical management is indicated for structural joint anomalies and palatal cleft. Intellect is normal.

Differential Diagnosis: Joint dislocations occur in **Hajdu-Cheney syndrome, otopalatodigidtal syndrome,** and **Ehlers-Danlos syndrome.** These syndromes have many other findings inconsistent with Larsen syndrome, including cognitive impairment (**otopalatodigital**), lax skin (**Ehlers-Danlos**), and dental anomalies (**Hajdu-Cheney**).

Lenz-Majewski Syndrome

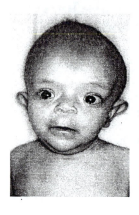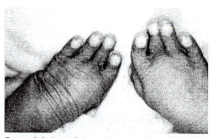

Lenz-Majewski syndrome: Characteristic facial appearance with associated digital anomalies including reduced length of the fingers.

Also Known As: Lenz-Majewski hyperostotic dwarfism.

This unusual syndrome of short stature and mental retardation is rare, but distinct. Almost all children with this syndrome are severely retarded.

Major System(s) Affected: Growth; craniofacial; limbs; musculoskeletal; central nervous system; dental; integument.

Etiology: Autosomal dominant expression is presumed, but has not been confirmed.

Quick Clues: The digital anomalies of Lenz-Majewski syndrome are distinctive and essentially unique.

Hearing Disorders: Sensorineural hearing loss is common.

Speech Disorders: Speech does not develop in many patients, or is severely limited in others.

Feeding Disorders: Early feeding may be severely impaired because of upper airway obstruction related to choanal atresia.

Voice Disorders: Voice disorders have not been observed or reported.

Resonance Disorders: Resonance disorders have not been observed or reported.

Language Disorders: Language is severely impaired, and in some cases, little useful language is acquired.

Other Clinical Features:

Growth: short stature;

Craniofacial: orbital hypertelorism; large appearing neurocranium; prolonged patency of the fontanels; prominent scalp veins; large appearing mouth; choanal atresia;

Limbs: reduced finger length; hypoplastic long bones;

Musculoskeletal: rib and clavicular hyperostoses;

Central nervous system: mental retardation, often severe;

Dental: enamel hypoplasia;

Integument: loose, thin, wrinkled skin.

Natural History: Birthweight is low, and growth deficiency becomes progressive after birth. The head appears large in infancy. The fontanels remain patent into childhood. Developmental delay is obvious in infancy.

Treatment Prognosis: Poor because of irreversible nature of the skeletal dysplasia and the severity of cognitive impairment.

Differential Diagnosis: The large neurocranium and patent fontanels are similar to the craniofacial manifestations seen in **cleidocranial dysplasia.** The developmental delay in Lenz-Majewski syndrome is not consistent with the developmental pattern in **cleidocranial dysplasia.**

L

Mannosidosis

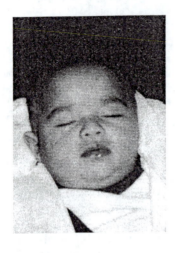

Mannosidosis: Mild coarsening of the face in an infant with mannosidosis.

Also Known As: Alpha-mannosidosis; alpha-mannosidase B deficiency.

Mannosidosis is another of the lysosomal storage diseases, similar in some ways to **Hurler, Hunter, Sanfilippo,** and **Morquio syndromes.** As in other lysosomal disorders, absence of a particular enzyme (in this case alpha-mannosidase) prevents the degradation of glycoproteins in the intracellular structures known as lysosomes. The glycoproteins are stored in the cells, thus distorting the cells and their functions. As with other lysosomal disorders, there is more than one form of the disease, a severe form with early onset (type I) and a milder form with late onset (type II).

Major System(s) Affected: Growth; central nervous system; craniofacial; musculoskeletal; hematologic; respiratory; immunologic, ocular.

Etiology: Autosomal recessive inheritance. The gene has been mapped to chromosome 19, at 19cen-q12 (from the centromere to the q12 band on the long arm of chromsome 19).

Quick Clues: Thickening of large auricles should be apparent by the time hearing is tested for a suspected hearing loss.

Hearing Disorders: In type II, high frequency sensorineural hearing loss is very common.

Speech Disorders: Infants with type I do not develop speech. Individuals with type II have delayed onset of speech. They tend to have sluggish articulation secondary to macroglossia and cognitive impairment. Dental spacing problems also lead to articulatory distortions.

Feeding Disorders: Infants with type I have failure-to-thrive secondary to severe neurologic impairment and chronic upper airway obstruction. In type II, feeding may be complicated by chronic congestion.

Voice Disorders: Voice is hoarse and wet secondary to chronic congestion and thickening of the vocal cord mucosa.

Resonance Disorders: Hyponasality is common secondary to chronic nasal congestion. The sensorineural hearing loss may contribute to the abnormal oral and nasal resonance patterns that accompany this type of hearing impairment.

Language Disorders: Infants with type I do not live long enough to develop language. In type II, language is essentially always delayed and impaired, but most individuals do obtain adequate language for communication.

Other Clinical Features:

Growth: tall stature;

Central nervous system: mental retardation; dilated ventricles; ataxia;

Craniofacial: coarse facial features; macrocephaly; thickened calvarium; low anterior hairline; thick, flat nose; macroglossia; gingival hypertrophy; mandibular prognathism; dental spacing; large, thick ears; bushy eyebrows;

Musculoskeletal: hypotonia; pectus carinatum; spondylosis;

Hematologic: abnormal lymphocytes; pancytopenia;

Respiratory: chronic upper and lower respiratory infections; chronic otitis;

Immunologic: immunoglobulin deficiency; hypogammaglobulinemia;

Ocular: corneal opacities.

Natural History: Newborns with type I do not survive infancy. The survival for type II is more favorable, but the onset of cognitive impairment and delayed development is early. The disorder is progressive, as are all lysosomal storage diseases.

Treatment Prognosis: Bone marrow transplantation has been suggested as being of possible benefit to patients with mannosidosis. However, no specific benefit of treatment has been demonstrated to date. Palliative treatment is certainly indicated.

Differential Diagnosis: Although the general features of all lysosomal storage diseases are similar, the diagnosis of the specific disorder is based on appropriate biochemical tests.

Marfan Syndrome

Also Known As:

Marfan syndrome is a well-recognized syndrome of connective tissue abnormalities that results in multiple skeletal and joint abnormalities. Marfan syndrome probably has a population prevalence of approximately 1:10,000.

Major System(s) Affected:
Musculoskeletal; ocular; craniofacial; cardiac; pulmonary.

Etiology: Autosomal dominant inheritance. Most cases are familial, but approximately 20% are new mutations. The gene has been mapped to 15q21.1 and has been identified as the fibrillin gene.

Quick Clues: Individuals with Marfan syndrome are typically tall and gangly with fingers that appear long and are hyperextensible. A vertically long face is also typical.

Hearing Disorders: Sensorineural hearing loss is not a common finding, but has been observed in some cases.

Speech Disorders: Articulation impairment is common secondary to malocclusion resulting in obligatory substitutions and distortions. Malocclusions typically involve vertical maxillary excess, maxillary constriction, dental crowding, and anterior skeletal open-bite. The dentofacial abnormalities are progressive. Therefore, articulation impairment often involves lingual protrusion.

Feeding Disorders: Feeding in infancy is usually normal. Later in life, malocclusion may lead to some chewing difficulties.

Voice Disorders: Hoarse voice is an occasional finding related to pulmonary disease.

Resonance Disorders: Resonance is typically normal.

Language Disorders: Language development is normal, as is cognition.

Other Clinical Features:

Musculoskeletal: tall, thin body with disproportionately long limbs (known as marfanoid habitus); scoliosis or kyphoscoliosis; pectus carinatum or excavatum; joint laxity; joint contractures; arachnodactyly;

Ocular: ectopia lentis (dislocated lens); myopia; retinal detachment;

Craniofacial: dolicocephaly; vertical maxillary excess with "long face"; anterior skeletal open-bite, vertical growth pattern; dental crowding;

Cardiac: aortic aneurysm; aortic dissection; aortic regurgitation; mitral valve prolapse; aortic root dilation; right-sided heart enlargement and congestive heart failure;

Pulmonary: restrictive pulmonary disease; emphysema; pneumothorax; pulmonary blebs.

Natural History: The facial and skeletal manifestations of Marfan syndrome are progressive, but typically become evident early in life. The cardiac and vascular anomalies may arise at any time, but sudden death secondary to aortic dissection is most common in early adult years. Early death is common. Cognition and overall development are normal.

Treatment Prognosis: Careful follow-up of cardiac status, especially aortic anomalies, is extremely important. Early management of scoliosis and spinal anomalies is also recommended to avoid pulmonary restriction. Increased intracardiac pressures can further exacerbate aortic dissections so that maintaining normal pulmonary capacity is important.

Differential Diagnosis: Joint hyperextensibility associated with myopia and "marfanoid habitus" may be observed in **Stickler syndrome.** Cleft palate, common in **Stickler syndrome,** does not occur in Marfan syndrome.

Maroteaux-Lamy Syndrome

Also Known As: Mucopolysaccharidosis type VI; arylsulfatase B deficiency.

Maroteaux-Lamy syndrome has three subtypes: mild, moderate, and severe. In all three types, unlike many of the lysosomal storage diseases, cognitive abilities are normal in almost all cases. However, coarsening of the face and short stature are consistent findings. The syndrome is rare and does not occur in more than 1:100,000 births.

Major System(s) Affected: Craniofacial; growth; ocular; cardiopulmonary; musculoskeletal; abdominal/gut.

Etiology: Autosomal recessive inheritance. The gene has been mapped to 5q11-q13.

Quick Clues: Joint stiffness may be noticed in association with coarsening of the face.

Hearing Disorders: Both conductive and sensorineural hearing losses have been observed, but are not necessarily common manifestations of the syndrome.

Speech Disorders: Speech development is often normal initially, but articulation may become impaired secondary to enlargement of the tongue and eventual malocclusion, related to dental eruption problems secondary to thickened gingiva and alveolar bone abnormalities.

Feeding Disorders: Feeding is typically normal. Later in life, enlargement of the tongue and dental eruption abnormalities may cause some difficulty with chewing large or tough pieces of food.

Voice Disorders: Hoarseness is common secondary to mucosal thickening and chronic mucus build-up in the upper and lower airway.

Resonance Disorders: Resonance is initially normal, but with age and progression of the phenotype, hyponasality may occur secondary to chronic nasal congestion, especially in the most severe cases. Oral resonance may also be abnormal secondary to thickening of the tongue, oral mucosa, and tonsils.

M

Language Disorders: Language development is almost always normal.

Other Clinical Features:

Craniofacial: coarse facial appearance; enlarged tongue; thickened maxillary and mandibular alveolus; dental spacing anomalies; dental eruption anomalies; thickened palate and buccal surfaces; thickened mucosa;

Growth: short stature;

Ocular: corneal opacities;

Cardiopulmonary: valve anomalies; chronic upper and lower airway disease; pulmonary insufficiency;

Musculoskeletal: joint stiffness; lumbar kyphosis; genu valgum; hip dysplasia; pectus carinatum;

Abdominal/gut: inguinal hernia; hepatosplenomegaly.

Natural History: The age of onset varies for the three subtypes. In the mildest form, onset is usually in childhood at about school age, while in the milder form, onset is in infancy. In all subtypes, cognition is normal, but the other findings vary in severity.

Treatment Prognosis: There is no known treatment for the progressive nature of the anomalies. In the mildest form, patients survive to adult years. In the most severe form, premature death may occur in adolescence or late childhood, caused by the combined effects of heart valve abnormalities and pulmonary disease.

Differential Diagnosis: The coarsening facial features and growth deficiency are nearly consistent findings in the majority of the lysosomal storage diseases. The differentiation is made by laboratory tests.

Marshall Syndrome

Also Known As:

Marshall syndrome is a disorder that has been regarded to be clinically similar to **Stickler syndrome,** and in the past, many clinicians believed that **Stickler syndrome** and Marshall syndrome were simply variable expressions of the same disorder. Some clinicians called both disorders the Marshall-Stickler syndrome. However, it now seems apparent that **Stickler syndrome** and Marshall syndrome are separate disorders with **Stickler** being a far more common form of connective tissue dysplasia.

Major System(s) Affected:
Craniofacial; integument; ocular.

Etiology:
Autosomal dominant inheritance. The gene has been mapped to 1p21 and has been identified as a collagen gene, *COL11A1.*

Quick Clues:
A child presenting with thick glasses (indicative of high myopia) and a round face with hypertelorism should be suspected of having Marshall syndrome or one of the similar connective tissue dysplasias.

Hearing Disorders:
Sensorineural hearing loss occurs in a high percentage of patients with Marshall syndrome. The loss is typically high frequency and may be progressive.

Speech Disorders:
Articulation may be impaired by malocclusion, including a Class II relationship with open-bite, and constriction of the maxillary arch. Compensatory articulation patterns occur secondary to cleft palate and velopharyngeal insufficiency.

Feeding Disorders:
Upper airway obstruction is a possible finding in Marshall syndrome that may interfere with infant feeding.

Voice Disorders:
Voice is normal.

Resonance Disorders:
Hypernasal resonance occurs in some cases with cleft palate. However, nasal obstruction secondary to a small nasal capsule and a small nasopharynx may also occur.

Language Disorders:
Language and cognition are usually normal.

M

Other Clinical Features:

Craniofacial: maxillary deficiency; cleft palate; mild micrognathia; hypertelorism; thickening of the neurocranium;

Integument: patches of cutis aplasia;

Ocular: high myopia; cataracts; glaucoma; strabismus; retinal detachment possible with age.

Natural History: At birth, some babies with Marshall syndrome present with Robin sequence, but this association is not as frequent as with **Stickler syndrome.** Midfacial deficiency becomes evident with age, but is not apparent in infancy. However, the malocclusion often remains Class II with a maxillary overjet because the mandible may be hypoplastic as well. Myopia is often present and severe at birth and becomes progressively worse with age. Hearing loss may be mildly progressive.

Treatment Prognosis: The prognosis is excellent. Cognition is normal. Myopia can be managed with spectacles and eventually with surgery, as can retinal detachment. Speech outcome from surgical repair of the palate is usually excellent.

Differential Diagnosis: Stickler syndrome has a very similar phenotype, but without the cutis aplasia or calvarial thickening. **Stickler syndrome** also has joint abnormalities and epiphyseal dysplasia.

Michels Syndrome

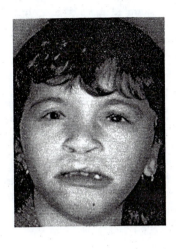

Michels syndrome: Note the bilateral cleft lip and palate and blepharophimosis in an eight-year-old girl with Michels syndrome.

Also Known As: Oculopalato-skeletal syndrome.

Although this syndrome is reportedly rare, it is likely that it is under-diagnosed because of the association of cleft lip and palate with conductive hearing loss, which is a common association in nonsyndromic clefting. In Michels syndrome, the conductive hearing loss is more severe than one would expect to find with chronic middle ear effusion and is likely to be related to ossicular anomalies, such as fusions or malformations.

Major System(s) Affected: Craniofacial; ocular; musculoskeletal; central nervous system.

Etiology: Autosomal recessive inheritance. The gene has not been mapped or identified.

Quick Clues: Blepharophimosis is an easily noticed anomaly of the inner canthi of the eyes that limits the palpebral fissure length. When found in association with cranial asymmetry and conductive hearing loss, Michels syndrome should be suspected.

M

Hearing Disorders: Conductive hearing loss in the moderate to severe range has been documented.

Speech Disorders: Speech is delayed and impaired, secondary both to cleft palate and cognitive impairment.

Feeding Disorders: Early feeding may be problematic secondary to cleft palate and central nervous system impairment resulting in hypertonicity.

Voice Disorders: Voice disorders have not been noted or reported.

Resonance Disorders: Hypernasality secondary to cleft palate is likely.

Language Disorders: Language impairment is common secondary to cognitive impairment and some degree of contribution of conductive hearing loss.

Other Clinical Features:

> **Craniofacial:** cleft lip-cleft palate; craniosynostosis; cranial asymmetry; blepharophimosis with shortened palpebral fissures;

> **Ocular:** corneal opacities; limited upward gaze; ptosis;

> **Musculoskeletal:** radioulnar synostosis; spina bifida occulta; short fifth finger with single flexion crease;

> **Central nervous system:** developmental delay; cognitive impairment (mild); infantile hypertonicity.

Natural History: The anomalies in Michels syndrome are congenital and static without progression, including the hearing loss.

Treatment Prognosis: The prognosis is good with the structural anomalies amenable to surgical reconstruction. Hearing loss responds well to amplification and may be treated surgically as well.

Differential Diagnosis: Blepharophimosis syndrome does not have cleft lip and palate as a feature, but not all patients with Michels syndrome have facial clefts. **Ohdo syndrome** also has blepharophimosis as a feature. Several of the **oral-facial-digital syndromes** and **craniofrontonasal syndrome** have cleft lip and palate as common features with laterally displaced inner canthi.

Miller Syndrome

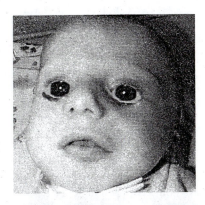

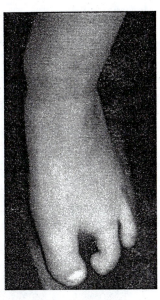

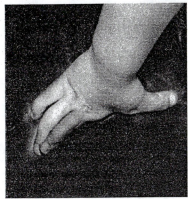

Miller syndrome: An infant with Miller syndrome showing ectropion of the lower eyelids. The foot shows absence of the second and third toes and the hand also has a missing postaxial digit and hypoplastic thumb.

Also Known As: Gené-Wiedemann syndrome; POADS.

Miller syndrome resembles **Treacher Collins syndrome** with abnormalities of the lower eyelids and cleft palate or cleft lip and palate and anomalous external ears. Miller syndrome differs from both **Treacher Collins syndrome** and **Nager syndrome** in relation to digital anomalies, specifically the presence of postaxial absence of digits on both the hands and feet.

Major System(s) Affected:
Craniofacial; musculoskeletal; gastrointestinal; genitourinary.

Etiology:
Autosomal recessive inheritance. The gene has not been mapped or identified.

Quick Clues:
A deep depression of the lower eyelids associated with absence of the fifth fingers is nearly pathognomonic for Miller syndrome.

Hearing Disorders:
Variable conductive hearing loss ranging from mild to severe is probably related to ossicular anomalies in the majority of cases. The external auditory canals are also stenotic in many cases.

Speech Disorders:
Speech may be impaired by clefting of the palate or lip and palate. Retrognathia may also result in malocclusion and its resulting obligatory articulation errors.

Feeding Disorders:
Feeding may be impaired in infancy secondary to airway obstruction from micrognathia and Robin sequence.

Voice Disorders:
Voice disorders have not been observed or reported.

Resonance Disorders:
Abnormal resonance is often present. In some cases, resonance is hypernasal secondary to clefting. In other cases, there is muffled oral resonance secondary to micrognathia and glossoptosis.

Language Disorders:
Language development is typically normal.

Other Clinical Features:

Craniofacial: lower eyelid ectropion; cleft palate or cleft lip and palate; cup-shaped ears; malar deficiency; micrognathia;

Musculoskeletal: ulnar hypoplasia or aplasia; radioulnar synostosis; absence of the fifth fingers and metacarpals; hypoplastic thumbs; short forearms; hypoplastic/aplastic second and third toes;

Gastrointestinal: malrotation of the gut;

Genitourinary: renal anomalies;

Other: supernumerary nipples.

Natural History: The anomalies associated with Miller syndrome are all congenital and nonprogressive.

Treatment Prognosis: Surgical reconstruction for the facial and hand anomalies is possible. Cognitive development is normal.

Differential Diagnosis: Miller syndrome resembles **Treacher Collins syndrome** and **Nager syndrome.** The anomalies associated with **Treacher Collins syndrome** are essentially isolated to the craniofacial complex, whereas Miller syndrome has characteristic limb anomalies. **Nager syndrome** has hypoplastic or absent thumbs, as does Miller syndrome, as well as possible radial-ulnar synostosis. Miller syndrome may be differentiated from **Nager syndrome** based on the ectropion of the lower eyelids.

Mohr Syndrome

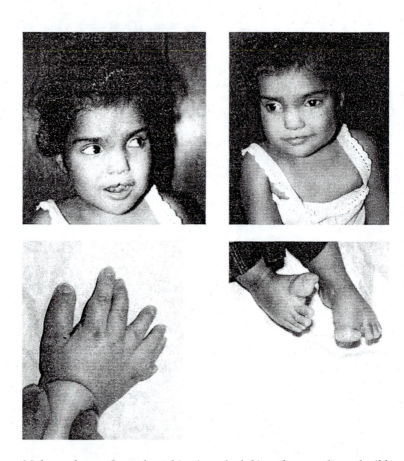

Mohr syndrome: Central notching (pseudocleft) on the upper lip and mild hypertelorism (top row) associated with polydactyly (bottom row) in Mohr syndrome (OFD type II).

Also Known As: Oral-facial-digital syndrome, type II; OFD II.

Mohr syndrome is one of the multiple anomaly disorders that have been classified as **oral-facial-digital syndromes.** The label oral-facial-digital does not connote any genetic or etiologic common ground, but rather is a descriptive nosological term based on several of the major clinical findings. The syndrome is rare with a population frequency of 1:300,000.

Major System(s) Affected: Craniofacial; growth; central nervous system; limbs.

Etiology: Autosomal recessive inheritance. The gene has not been mapped or identified.

Quick Clues: The presence of polydactyly associated with a midline cleft or notch of the lip should always raise the suspicion of Mohr syndrome or one of the other **oral-facial-digital syndromes.**

Hearing Disorders: Conductive hearing loss secondary to ossicular malformation, particularly of the incus, is common.

Speech Disorders: Speech is delayed in many cases, especially those with more significant cognitive impairment. Articulation is typically impaired secondary to lingual abnormalities, including a lobulated tongue and hamartomas of the tongue. A midline cleft of the lip also makes bilabial sound production difficult. Compensatory articulation patterns secondary to cleft palate and velopharyngeal insufficiency may also occur.

Feeding Disorders: Feeding may be complicated by newborn tachypnea.

Voice Disorders: Voice is typically normal.

Resonance Disorders: Hypernasal resonance secondary to cleft palate may occur.

Language Disorders: Language impairment is constant in those patients with cognitive impairment and central nervous system anomalies. In the most severe cases, there is limited language development.

Other Clinical Features:

> **Craniofacial:** Midline cleft lip; cleft palate; lobulated or cleft tongue; lingual hamartomas; abnormal cranial sutures;

Growth: short stature;

Central nervous system: cognitive impairment; cerebellar anomalies;

Limbs: polydactyly; syndactyly.

Natural History: All of the anomalies associated with Mohr syndrome are present at birth and are essentially static.

Treatment Prognosis: The prognosis depends on the degree of cognitive impairment and CNS anomalies. Some individuals with Mohr syndrome have died in childhood secondary to respiratory infections.

Differential Diagnosis: Digital and craniofacial anomalies are common features in all the **oral-facial digital syndromes.** Midline cleft lip is common in the premaxilary agenesis type of **holoprosencephaly.**

Morquio Syndrome

Also Known As: Mucopolysaccharidosis (MPS) type IV; galactosamine-6-sulfatase deficiency.

Morquio syndrome is another autosomal recessive lysosomal storage disease with a progressive course, but longer survival than **Hunter, Hurler,** or **Sanfilippo syndromes.** Also somewhat different from the other mucopolysaccharidoses, there is little, if any, facial coarsening in Morquio syndrome, with more of the effects being seen in the extracranial skeleton. Two subtypes have been described, a severe form labeled as MPS IVA and a mild, late onset type labeled MPS IVB. However, individuals clinically diagnosed with MPS IVB do not have galactosamine-6-sulfatase deficiency, indicating that the disorder is etiologically and genetically different from classic Morquio syndrome.

Major System(s) Affected: Growth; musculoskeletal; ocular; gastrointestinal; cardiopulmonary.

Etiology: Autosomal recessive inheritance. The gene has been mapped to 16q24.3 and has been labeled *GALNS*.

Quick Clues: The association of short stature with kyphoscoliosis should raise the suspicion of Morquio syndrome.

Hearing Disorders: Conductive hearing loss secondary to chronic middle ear effusion and "glue ear" is common.

Speech Disorders: Speech is essentially normal, but there is relative prognathism in some cases that may result in distortion of anterior sound production.

Feeding Disorders: Feeding is typically normal.

Voice Disorders: Voice is typically high-pitched and hoarse in adolescent and adult years.

Resonance Disorders: There is an unusual oropharyngeal resonance related to a short neck and limited resonating cavity. In adult years, persistent hyponasality is common secondary to chronic nasal congestion and obstruction.

M

Language Disorders: Language development and intellect are normal.

Other Clinical Features:

> **Growth:** short stature (average adult height is approximately three feet);

> **Musculoskeletal:** kyphoscoliosis; hip dysplasia; pectus carinatum; platyspondyly (flat vertebrae); atlanto-axial instability caused by a hypoplastic odontoid process that may result in spinal cord and nerve compression; joint laxity; genu valgum; thickened calvarial bones; increased space between the vertebrae; wide metaphyses; osteoporosis;

> **Ocular:** corneal opacities;

> **Gastrointestinal:** inguinal hernias; umbilical hernia; liver enlargement;

> **Cardiopulmonary:** valve anomalies; aortic regurgitation; restrictive pulmonary disease (secondary to skeletal anomalies).

Natural History: The onset of noticeable physical findings in Morquio syndrome is at approximately two years. Progression of respiratory symptoms and hearing loss is relatively slow compared to other lysosomal storage diseases. Most patients live into adult years, usually to the 20s or 30s, but complications of pulmonary restriction and possible spinal injury can complicate the prognosis and cause earlier death.

Treatment Prognosis: The long-term prognosis is poor, but palliative treatment in early life for middle ear disease is effective.

Differential Diagnosis: Morquio syndrome does not have the same facial phenotype as the other mucopolysaccharidoses, but the extracranial findings are similar. Also, unlike other mucopolysaccharidoses, intellect and behavior are normal. Severe kyphoscoliosis and short stature are common in diastrophic dysplasia and flattened vertebrae may be found in **spondyloepiphyseal dysplasia congenita.** However, the overall pattern of skeletal dysplasias in these syndromes is different and there are no signs of metabolic disease as in Morquio syndrome.

Multiple Lentigines Syndrome

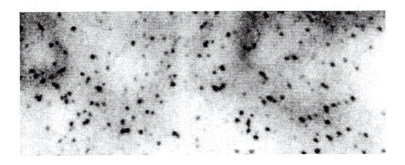

Multiple lentigines syndrome: Appearance of the skin showing multiple lentigines, small darkly pigmented growths.

Also Known As: LEOPARD syndrome; lentiginosis, cardiomyopathy.

This syndrome was first idenitifed as LEOPARD syndrome, an acronym for multiple *L*entigines, *E*lectrocardiographic conduction abnormalities, *O*cular hypertelorism, *P*ulmonic stenosis, *A*bnormal genitalia, *R*etarded growth, and sensorineural *D*eafness. The acronym is an attempt at humor because dark lentigines are distributed in many places on the body making individuals appear spotted like a leopard. Cutaneous abnormalities associated with cognitive impairments and hearing loss are common among other syndromes (such as neurofibromatosis and basal cell nevus syndrome) so that obvious pigmentary abnormalities should always raise an index of suspicion with the observant clinician.

Major System(s) Affected: Integument; cardiopulmonary; genitourinary; growth/endocrine; craniofacial.

Etiology: Autosomal dominant inheritance. The gene has not been mapped or identified.

Quick Clues: The patterns of densely grouped small dark birth marks are distinctive and easily visible in most patients.

Hearing Disorders: Mild sensorineural hearing loss is a common, but not consistent, feature of the syndrome. Several cases have been known to have more severe hearing loss. Vestibular abnormalities have not been found.

Speech Disorders: Speech and articulation are typically normal. However, there have been a number of cases with relatively large growths on the hard or soft palate that could interfere with tongue placement for articulation. In cases with severe or profound hearing loss (unusual), speech production will be severely impaired.

Feeding Disorders: Feeding is normal.

Voice Disorders: Voice production is normal.

Resonance Disorders: Resonance abnormalities have not been reported or observed except in relation to sensorineural deafness.

Language Disorders: Language is mildly impaired in many cases secondary to cognitive impairment.

Other Clinical Features:

    Integument: multiple small lentigines on the skin, not the mucous membranes; café-au-lait spots; occasional neoplasias;

    Cardiopulmonary: valvular pulmonic stenosis; cardiomyopathy; ECG abnormalities;

    Genitourinary: hypoplastic/aplastic ovaries; cryptorchidism; hypospadias;

    Growth/endocrine: short stature; late onset of puberty;

    Craniofacial: ocular hypertelorism.

Natural History: The lentigines are typically present at birth and increase in number with age. The heart and hearing anomalies may not be obvious, but are present at birth. Growth deficiency is of postnatal onset.

Treatment Prognosis: All disorders can be treated symptomatically with the prognosis being based on the severity.

Differential Diagnosis: Basal cell nevus syndrome has a similar appearance of the skin, but the other anomalies are not similar. The association of the heart and genitourinary problems make this diagnosis distinctive.

Nager Syndrome

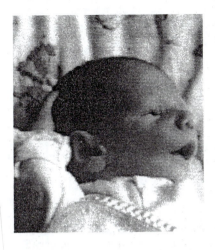
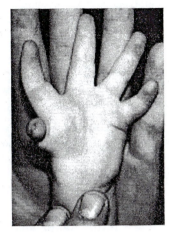

Nager syndrome: Severe micrognathia, Robin sequence, and hypoplasia of the thumb in an infant with Nager syndrome.

Also Known As: Acrofacial dysostosis; acrofacial dysostosis 1, Nager type; preaxial acrofacial dysostosis.

Nager syndrome is a rare craniofacial disorder that closely resembles **Treacher Collins syndrome,** but has the added finding of radial and hand anomalies. The syndrome has some striking findings, including severe micrognathia and severe hypoplasia of the soft palate. The author has seen several cases with little more than a uvula extending from the hard palate.

Major System(s) Affected: Craniofacial; limbs.

Etiology: The etiology of Nager syndrome has been debated since the disorder was first recognized. Autosomal recessive and autosomal dominant inheritance have both been proposed, but the majority of cases have been sporadic. Recessive inheritance seems likely with several instances of affected siblings with normal parents having been observed. Etiologic heterogeneity has not been ruled out.

Quick Clues: Hypoplastic or absent thumbs associated with microtia is a strong indication for the diagnosis of Nager syndrome.

Hearing Disorders: Conductive hearing loss is a nearly constant finding, and is often maximal with ossicular malformations, variable microtia, and fixation of the footplate of the stapes.

Speech Disorders: Articulation disorders are a nearly constant finding in Nager syndrome. Unusually severe micrognathia leads to Class II occlusal relationships, openbite, and limited oral opening. The tongue is often quite small, but still has difficulty maneuvering in a small oral cavity. Tongue-backing is a common articulatory maneuver leading to very abnormal substitutions that are probably obligatory in nature. Cleft palate is common, and the cleft is often very severe, resulting in compensatory patterns that include tongue backing, glottal stops, pharyngeal stops, and laryngeal stops.

Feeding Disorders: Early failure-to-thrive secondary to airway obstruction is very common. Tracheotomy is often necessary in Nager syndrome because of the severity of micrognathia. Robin sequence is a common secondary disorder in Nager syndrome.

Voice Disorders: Voice is typically normal.

Resonance Disorders: Resonance is almost always anomalous with abnormalities of both oral and nasal resonance. Nasal resonance may be either hyponasal (if the palate is intact) or hypernasal (if the palate is cleft). In some cases, there is mixed hyper/hyponasality. Some patients with clefts have almost no soft palate with the uvula extending off the hard palate with little intervening tissue. In such cases, palate reconstruction becomes extremely difficult and may require pharyngeal flap. However, because of the potential for airway obstruction, pharyngeal flap may not be possible without some advancement of the mandible. Oral resonance is usually very muffled because of posterior positioning of the tongue. In cases where the palate is cleft, the combination of muffled oral resonance with velopharyngeal insufficiency yields a very abnormal and unusual resonance pattern.

Language Disorders: Language development is typically normal and intellect is typically normal.

Other Clinical Features:

    Craniofacial: micrognathia, usually severe; cleft palate; microtia; ossicular anomalies; downslanting eyes; lower lid depressions; absent eyelashes of the inner third of the eye; zygomatic hypoplasia or clefting; acute flexion of the cranial base;

    Limbs: radial hypoplasia; absent or hypoplastic thumbs; radio-ulnar synsotosis; decreased extension of elbows.

Natural History: All the anomalies associated with Nager syndrome are present at birth and are nonprogressive. A pectus excavatum may develop because of upper airway obstruction, resulting in negative pressure and rib cage distortion. There is no "catch-up" growth of the mandible with age.

Treatment Prognosis: The severity of the craniofacial anomalies in Nager syndrome make early reconstruction difficult. The severe deficiency of tissue in the palate will often prevent early palate repair. Mandibular distraction may have significant advantages in Nager syndrome because of the severity of the mandibular deficiency. Because failure-to-thrive is related to airway obstruction, treatment of obstructive apnea should be aggressive prior to recommending alternative feeding procedures.

Differential Diagnosis: Nager syndrome is almost identical to **Treacher Collins syndrome** in relation to the craniofacial findings, but **Treacher Collins syndrome** does not have limb anomalies as a clinical finding.

N

Neurofibromatosis, Type 2

Also Known As: NF2.

Neurofibromatosis, type 2, is less common than the more familiar type 1 that is often referred to as von Recklinhausen disease. However, the recognition that acoustic nerve tumors occur in neurofibromatosis was based on the observation of type 2 cases. Acoustic neuroma is not a feature of NF1, but is a major finding in NF2.

Major System(s) Affected: Integument; craniofacial; central nervous system; ocular; skeletal; cardiac.

Etiology: Autosomal dominant inheritance. The gene has been mapped to 22q12.2. The NF2 gene is a type of tumor suppressor gene. Multiple mutations have been found in individuals with NF2, the net effect being the truncation of the protein normally encoded by the NF2 gene. The effect is the formation of various types of auditory tumors, including schwannomas.

Speech Disorders: Speech onset is often delayed. Mild dysar-thria has been observed. Impaired articulation secondary to malocclusion and facial weakness is also found.

Feeding Disorders: Feeding disorders have not been a common observation.

Hearing Disorders: Hearing loss is present in about half of all cases, 75% being unilateral. The hearing loss is neural or central. Vestibular function is impaired.

Voice Disorders: Voice is normal.

Resonance Disorders: Hypernasality secondary to asymmetric movement of the velopharyngeal valve has been observed in some older patients.

Language Disorders: Language development is initially normal.

Other Clinical Features:

> **Integument:** several café-au-lait macules may be found, but not as many as in NF1.

Small pigmented neurofibromas are also found.

Craniofacial: facial tumors; facial asymmetry; facial weakness.

Central nervous system: macrencephaly; learning disorders; seizures; meningiomas, ataxia, gliomas.

Ocular: optic nerve glioma; Lisch nodules; glaucoma; ptosis; corneal opacity;

Other: various tumors may develop, including some malignancies.

Natural History: At birth, there may be no sign of anomalies. Usually the first presentation is the café-au-lait macules with tumors developing later in life. Life expectancy may be decreased in some cases secondary to tumor formation, occasional malignancy, or complications from benign growths. Hearing loss usually develops in adolescent years, sometimes later. Effects of CNS or peripheral tumors are progressive. The first signs of hearing loss may be discrimination disorders. The progressive effects of CNS tumors and increased intracranial pressure occurs in adult life, often in the 30s.

Treatment Prognosis: Fair to excellent depending on the type and location of tumors.

Differential Diagnosis: Café-au-lait spots may be found in over 100 genetic disorders. Abnormal tumor and hamartoma growth occurs in Proteus syndrome, Bannayan-Zonana syndrome, and Klippel-Trénaunay-Weber syndrome. Asymmetric craniofacial growth is found in hemihyperplasia and McCune-Albright syndrome.

N

Niikawa-Kuroki Syndrome

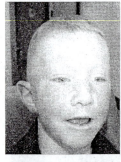
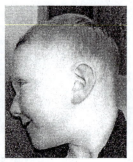
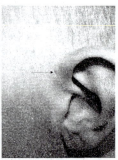

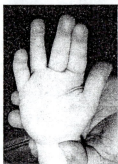

Niikawa-Kuroki syndrome: Note the wide palpebral fissures, large ears, preauricular pit (arrow at far right), and thickened finger pads in Niikawa-Kuroki syndrome.

Also Known As: Kabuki syndrome; Kabuki make-up syndrome.

Niikawa-Kuroki syndrome is most often referred to as Kabuki syndrome, a name initially coined based on facial appearance. The appearance of the eyes, with eversion of the lateral portion of the lids showing the red conjunctiva, gave the impression of the make-up worn by Kabuki theater performers in Japan. The use of the term "Kabuki," while not specifically meant to be humorous, has a connotation that can be interpreted as being pejorative because of the exaggerated make-up style of Kabuki performers. It is, therefore, preferred to use the eponym of Niikawa-Kuroki syndrome in honor of the scientists who initially described the syndrome. The incidence of the syndrome is not known in all populations, but an estimated 1:30,000 individuals are affected in Japan. The syndrome is probably equally common worldwide.

Quick Clues: Marked erythema of the face in a mask-like distribution. Also, the ear pit in Niikawa-Kuroki syndrome is in a distinctive location, similar to that of **BOR syndrome,** but different from that typically found in isolated examples or **oculo-auriculo-vertebral spectrum** disorder.

Major System(s) Affected: Craniofacial; central nervous system; growth; cardiac; limbs; musculoskeletal.

Etiology: Autosomal dominant inheritance. The gene has not been mapped or identified.

Hearing Disorders: Conductive hearing loss is common in infancy and childhood secondary to chronic otitis media. Malformed ossicles may also be found.

Speech Disorders: Many children with Niikawa-Kuroki syndrome develop only limited speech. Others have severe articulatory impairment related to cognitive impairment and hypotonia, as well as the secondary effects of cleft palate and velopharyngeal insufficiency leading to compensatory articulation.

Feeding Disorders: Early feeding is often problematic based on multiple causes. Congenital heart anomalies (often severe) and hypotonia (often severe) lead to early failure-to-thrive, and may result in the use of alternative feeding procedures, such as gavage feedings or gastrostomy.

Voice Disorders: Voice may be hoarse, or high pitched.

Resonance Disorders: Hypernasal resonance is common in cases with cleft palate which may, in part, be related to the hypotonia common in the syndrome.

Language Disorders: Language is essentially always impaired, and often severely impaired. The onset of first words is severely delayed in most cases, and other language milestones are also very delayed.

Other Clinical Features:

>**Craniofacial:** wide palpebral fissures; everted lateral

portions of the lower eyelids with conjunctival show; microcephaly; cleft palate; large ears with prominent ear lobes; open-mouth posture; wide nose with depressed nasal tip;

Central nervous system: mental retardation; seizures;

Growth: small stature;

Cardiac: conotruncal heart anomalies; aortic aneurysm; right bundle branch block; transposition of the great vessels; single ventricle;

Limbs: persistent fetal finger pads;

Musculoskeletal: scoliosis; spina bifida occulta; abnormal hip joints; rib anomalies.

Natural History: Early neonatal history is difficult because of the combined effects of congenital heart disease, hypotonia and neurologically based developmental impairment, and failure-to-thrive. Language milestones tend to be delayed and impaired more significantly than cognitive performance might predict. Small stature becomes apparent in infancy with postnatal growth deficiency.

Treatment Prognosis: Variable, depending on the degree of cognitive impairment. Although language and speech milestones seem to be disproportionately affected, treatment should be implemented as soon as possible and as vigorously as possible.

Differential Diagnosis: The association of conotruncal heart anomalies with cleft palate and hypotonia is common in **velo-cardiofacial syndrome (VCFS).** However, in **VCFS,** the ears are small with overfolded helices and absent lobules, whereas in Niikawa-Kuroki syndrome, the ears are large and the lobule prominent. Small stature, heart anomalies, and cleft palate may also be found in **fetal alcohol syndrome** (FAS), but in FAS, the palpebral fissures are short and the ears tend to be small.

Noonan Syndrome

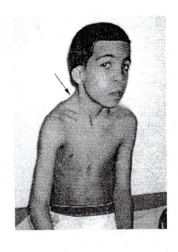

Noonan syndrome: Note pterygium colli (arrow) and low-set, posteriorly rotated ears in Noonan syndrome.

Also Known As: Pterygium colli syndrome.

Noonan syndrome is a disorder that bears a strong physical resemblance to **Turner syndrome,** but is not associated with a sex chromosome abnormality and is not limited to expression in females. It is one of the more common multiple anomaly syndromes with a population prevalence of approximately 1:2,500.

Major System(s) Affected: Craniofacial/head and neck; cardiac; central nervous system; growth; genitourinary; musculoskeletal; hematologic; integument.

Quick Clues: Webbing of the neck, although a feature of a number of other syndromes, should always raise the suspicion of a diagnosis of Noonan syndrome, especially in males. **Turner syndrome** also has webbing of the neck as a feature, but all patients with **Turner syndrome** are phenotypically female.

Etiology: Autosomal dominant inheritance. The gene has been mapped to 12q24.

N

Hearing Disorders: Conductive, sensorineural, and mixed hearing loss have all been observed in Noonan syndrome, but are relatively low frequency anomalies.

Speech Disorders: Speech is marked by many obligatory articulation errors related to malocclusion, including class II malocclusion, anterior skeletal open-bite, and a constricted maxillary arch. There is, in some patients, limitation of mandibular movement secondary to vertical maxillary excess and a steep mandibular plane angle. Cleft palate is a low frequency anomaly, and in most cases is submucous when present. Submucous cleft may lead to compensatory articulation patterns secondary to velopharyngeal insufficiency.

Feeding Disorders: Early feeding problems and failure-to-thrive are common, occurring in nearly half of cases. Feeding is complicated by airway obstruction, or by congenital heart disease, particularly pulmonary stenosis. Hypotonia is also present in approximately one-third of cases.

Voice Disorders: Voice is typically normal, but in some cases with more severe growth deficiency, it may be high-pitched.

Resonance Disorders: Resonance may be hypernasal in a small percentage of patients with Noonan syndrome secondary to cleft palate (usually submucous). Oral resonance is occasionally muffled because the neck may be shorter than normal, reducing the resonating volume of the oropharynx and hypopharynx.

Language Disorders: Language development is variable and is dependent on the presence of cognitive impairment. Intellect in Noonan syndrome ranges from mild mental retardation to superior intelligence, with approximately a third of cases showing some cognitive impairment. Language delay is common and has been attributed to perceptual-motor problems. Expressive language is usually proportionately more impaired than receptive. Learning disabilities have also been noted.

Other Clinical Features:

Craniofacial/head and neck: Webbing of the neck (pterygium colli); cervical hygroma; triangular facial contour; deep furrow in the philtrum; prominent cupid's bow; vertical maxillary excess; vertical facial growth pattern with steep mandibular plane; low-set ears; posteriorly rotated ears; low posterior hairline; ptosis; mild orbital hypertelorism, downslanting eyes; anterior skeletal open-bite; constricted maxillary arch;

Cardiac: pulmonary stenosis; pulmonary valve dysplasia; patent ductus arteriosus; coarctation of the aorta; cardiomyopathy;

Central nervous system: cognitive impairment; perceptual impairments; learning disabilities;

Growth: short stature;

Genitourinary: cryptorchidism; male infertility;

Musculoskeletal: pectus excavatum and/or carinatum; "shield-shaped" chest; cubitus valgus; short distal phalanges;

Hematologic/lymphatic: lymphedema; von Willebrand disease; thrombocytopenia;

Integument: cutaneous lymphangioma; tendency toward easy bruising;

Other: malignant schwannoma.

Natural History: Developmental delay is relatively mild in cases with cognitive impairment, but in those cases, speech tends to be disproportionately delayed and expressive language more significantly impaired than intellect would predict. Thrombocytopenia may not be noted until later in life. Lymphedema may be present early, and may even be detected prenatally using ultrasound. If the heart anomalies are not too severe, life expectancy may be normal, although some patients do develop malignancies. Some patients with severe heart anomalies have a shortened life span.

Treatment Prognosis: The prognosis for Noonan syndrome is dependent on the severity of the heart anomalies and cognitive status. In general, the speech, language, and learning disorders do respond favorably to traditional therapeutic approaches. The facial anomalies and malocclusion typically require surgical intervention in teen years. Therefore, speech therapy, though effective for the language disorders and speech delay, will have little or no impact on obligatory sound errors caused by malocclusion.

Differential Diagnosis: Webbing of the neck is common in **Turner syndrome,** but all **Turner** cases are phenotypically female and have an obvious karyotypic abnormality. The Noonan phenotype has also been observed in patients with **velo-cardio-facial syndrome (VCFS),** including webbing of the neck, cryptorchidism, learning disabilities; thrombocytopenia, pulmonary stenosis, short distal phalanges, and disproportionately delayed expressive language. However, learning and cognitive problems are more common in **VCFS,** and mental illness is a manifestation of **VCFS** that has not been reported as a manifestation of Noonan syndrome.

Norrie Syndrome

Also Known As: Norrie disease; atrophia bulborum hereditaria; pseudoglioma.

Norrie syndrome has been recognized as a diagnostic entity for nearly a century, with hundreds of cases having been described. It is an X-linked recessive disorder so that essentially all cases are male.

Major System(s) Affected: Ocular; central nervous system; genitourinary.

Etiology: X-linked recessive inheritance. The gene has been mapped to Xp11.4.

Quick Clues: Atrophy of the iris and congenital cataracts are easily visible to even casual observation.

Hearing Disorders: Moderate to severe sensorineural hearing loss is the rule, but mild and profound cases have been observed. Onset is typically in the early second decade of life and the course is progressive. The hearing loss is cochlear without retrocochlear components.

Speech Disorders: Speech begins to develop normally but may deteriorate later in life with the onset of progressive mental deterioration.

Feeding Disorders: Feeding disorders have not been reported or observed.

Voice Disorders: Voice disorders have not been reported or observed.

Resonance Disorders: Resonance is normal initially, but may become impaired secondary to the progressive hearing loss.

Language Disorders: Language development is initially normal in many cases, but may deteriorate with the onset of mental and cognitive impairment.

Other Clinical Features:

    Ocular: cataracts; iris atrophy; retinopathy; corneal degeneration;

    Central nervous system: primary microcephaly; cognitive impairment; cognitive degeneration; psychiatric illness; seizures;

Genitourinary: cryptorchidism; hypospadias.

Natural History: Cognitive deterioration and psychiatric problems vary in age at onset, based on the severity of expression. The more severe the disorder, the earlier the onset. In the most severe cases, the onset of mental deterioration occurs within the first few years of life. Blindness occurs in all cases and is congenital in many. Sensorineural hearing loss typically develops in the second decade of life and is progressive.

Treatment Prognosis: In the more severe cases with early onset of mental deterioration, the prognosis is poor. Blindness is universal, even when not congenital. Hearing loss is progressive, but may be successfully treated with amplification in the milder cases.

Differential Diagnosis: Congenital cataracts and corneal opacifications are found in **rubella embryopathy, cytomegalovirus embryopathy,** and **Harboyan syndrome.** However, the deterioration of central nervous system impairment is specific to Norrie syndrome.

Oculo-Auriculo-Vertebral Dysplasia (or Spectrum)

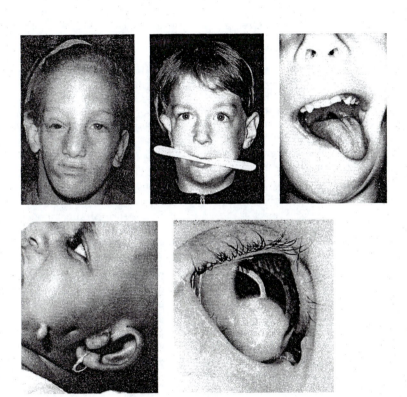

Oculo-auriculo-vertebral dysplasia: Note facial asymmetry, upward cant of the bite plane and asymmetric tongue movement (top row), ear tags and pits and ocular deremoid (bottom row).

Also Known As: Hemifacial microsomia; facio-auriculo-vertebral sequence; lateral facial dysplasia; Goldenhar syndrome; OAVS.

Oculo-auriculo-vertebral dysplasia (OAVS) is one of the most common craniofacial anomalies in man, perhaps second only to cleft palate as a type of craniofacial malformation. The population prevalence of the disorder is approximately 1:5,000. It is probable that an infant born with unilateral microtia has OAVS, unless the microtia is a feature of another syndrome such as **Treacher Collins syndrome.**

Major System(s) Affected: Craniofacial; ocular; musculoskeletal; central nervous system, cardiopulmonary.

Etiology: OAVS is etiologically heterogeneous. The disorder is not a specific syndrome, per se, but rather a developmental sequence that is presumed to be related to an embryonic vascular disruption in many cases. However, OAVS does occur as a secondary sequence in other syndromes and malformation sequences, including trisomy 18, del(18q), and **velo-cardio-facial syndrome.**

Quick Clues: Unilateral microtia, facial asymmetry (especially when accompanied by ear tags or pits), and ocular dermoid cysts should all point towards the possible diagnosis of OAVS, either singly or in combination.

Hearing Disorders: Conductive hearing loss, usually unilateral, is a nearly constant finding. Middle and external ear malformations may range from fixation of the footplate of the stapes to complete absence of the external and middle ear. Many cases of OAVS have bilateral manifestations so that conductive hearing loss may be bilateral, but asymmetric. Sensorineural components to the hearing loss have been observed in a small percentage of cases, including some cases with complete agenesis of the inner ear. The conductive hearing loss is often maximal, especially when accompanied by significant microtia.

Speech Disorders: Speech is delayed in many cases. Articulation impairment is very common with obligatory distortions and substitutions secondary to malocclusion, including lateral open-bites, anterior skeletal open-bites, micrognathia (unilateral or bilateral), unilateral paresis of the tongue and/or face; and missing dentition. Unilateral facial nerve paresis is common. Unilateral macrostomia is also common and may result in some distortions of sounds produced in the front of the oral cavity. Cleft lip and alveolus, a common malformation associated with OAVS, will also cause placement errors and distortions. Ankyloglossia caused by a short genioglossus muscle (often unilaterally) is also common. Compensatory articulation patterns secondary to cleft palate and velopharyngeal insufficiency are also common. Glossoptosis resulting in upper airway obstruction often results in fronting errors with lingual protrusion.

Feeding Disorders: Early feeding is frequently impaired and failure-to-thrive is a common early manifestation of OAVS. In nearly all cases, early feeding problems are related to airway obstruction. Unilateral hypoplasia of the pharynx and micrognathia combined with ankyloglossia results in upper airway obstruction and difficulty in coordinating breathing and eating. Many babies burn enormous amounts of calories just maintaining respiration and lose weight. When older, dental and occlusal anomalies may make chewing certain foods difficult. Feeding may also be complicated by some of the associated anomalies occasionally found in OAVS, including congeni-

tal heart disease, tracheoesophageal fistula, anal malformations, and pulmonary anomalies.

Voice Disorders: Hoarse or breathy voice secondary to unilateral vocal cord paresis is a common finding.

Resonance Disorders: Hypernasal resonance secondary to cleft palate is common, but hypernasality is also observed secondary to unilateral paresis and hypoplasia of the palate and/or pharynx. Asymmetric velopharyngeal insufficiency is a common manifestation of the syndrome and is actually more common than central velopharyngeal gaps, even in cases with cleft palate.

Language Disorders: Language development is typically normal, unless one of the associated findings is cognitive impairment. In some cases, cognitive impairment is severe and language does not develop, but these are unusual cases and are typically part of another syndrome complex that has OAVS as a secondary sequence.

Other Clinical Features:

> **Craniofacial:** unilateral or bilateral hypoplasia of the

mandible; absence of the condyle and/or coronoid (unilateral); absence or hypoplasia of the ramus (unilateral); facial nerve paresis; micrognathia; cleft palate; cleft lip and alveolus; preauricular skin tags and/or pits; cervical skin tags; microtia; anotia; ossicular malformations or aplasia; absence of the glenoid fossa (unilateral); macrostomia; lateral oral commissue cleft; cleft or absence of the zygoma (unilateral); lateral or anterior skeletal open-bite; shifting malocclusions; asymmetric movement of the palate and pharynx; unilateral hypoplasia of the pharynx or palate; hypoplasia or aplasia of the parotid glands; asymmetric cranium;

Ocular: clefts of the eyelids or orbits; microphthalmia; anophthalmia; dermoid cysts of the conjunctiva or limbus; orbital dystopia; strabismus;

Musculoskeletal: cervical spine anomalies; vertebral fusions; occipitalization of the atlas; Klippel-Feil anomaly; hemivertebrae; butterfly vertebrae; spina bifida occulta; scoliosis; rib anomalies;

club foot; occasional limb anomalies including thumb and radial malformations;

Central nervous system: occasional cognitive impairment; encephalocele; brain lipoma; Arnold-Chiari anomaly; **holoprosencephaly;** arachnoid cyst;

Cardiopulmonary: various heart malformations, including ventriculoseptal defect, tetralogy of Fallot, atrial septal defect; aplastic or hypoplastic lungs.

Natural History: Many infants with OAVS have severe airway obstruction at birth that may require tracheotomy. Failure-to-thrive should be a strong indication that airway obstruction is occurring, and prior to implementing operative approaches to feeding disorders (i.e., gastrostomy), the approach should be to resolve the airway obstruction. Tracheotomy is necessary in some cases. Conductive hearing loss is present from birth and hearing should therefore be assessed at the first possible sign of external ear anomalies or facial asymmetry. Cervical spine anomalies are also common and should be assessed immediately because hyperextension of the neck could result in damage to the spinal cord. Facial form and symmetry may be relatively normal at birth in milder cases, but with growth, the hypoplastic side becomes progressively smaller relative to the normal growing side. An upward cant to the bite plane develops and the occlusion may become unstable and shift because the lower arch does not match the upper arch. Compensatory downward overgrowth of the maxillary alveolus occurs on the side of the mandibular hypoplasia resulting in the canting of the bite plane. In the early teen years, the facial asymmetry becomes more pronounced because the normal side of the mandible undergoes its normal growth spurt while the hypoplastic side continues to lag.

Treatment Prognosis: In the absence of cognitive impairment, the prognosis is excellent because of the availability of excellent reconstructive procedures for the facial skeleton, the external ear, and the middle ear. Because the hearing loss is nearly always purely conductive, amplification can be successful in bringing hearing to normal limits; if there is bilateral loss, and with unilateral hearing loss, most affected individuals function very well with preferential seating in school. New reconstructive procedures, such as osseous distraction, can have a positive outcome in relation to facial asymmetry and airway obstruction.

Differential Diagnosis: Facial asymmetry with ear tags occurs in **Townes-Brocks syndrome** (commonly) and **velo-cardio-facial syndrome** (uncommonly). **BOR (branchi-oto-renal syndrome)** has the association of preauricular ear pits, dysmorphic ears, and hearing loss. Microtia, usually bilateral, with conductive hearing loss, cleft palate, occasional cleft lip, respiratory disorders, failure-to-thrive, and micrognathia occur in both **Treacher Collins syndrome** and **Nager syndrome,** and on occasion, these disorders can have mild facial asymmetry or ear tags. Cervical spine radiographs are certainly indicated when microtia occurs to help confirm the diagnosis with the added advantage of demonstrating potentially dangerous malformations of the cervical spine.

Oculo-Dento-Digital Syndrome

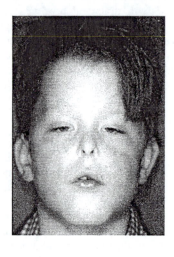

Oculo-dento-digital syndrome: Note the nasal alar hypoplasia.

Also Known As: Oculodento-osseous syndrome; oculodentodigital dysplasia.

Oculo-dento-digital syndrome (ODD) is a rare autosomal dominant disorder with a high spontaneous mutation rate. The combination of ocular, dental, and hand anomalies is distinctive and easily recognized. Performance and cognitive abilities are typically normal.

Major System(s) Affected: Ocular; dental; craniofacial; limbs; integument; neurologic.

Etiology: Autosomal dominant inheritance. The gene has been mapped to 6q22-q24.

Quick Clues: The association of small eyes with hypodontia and sparse scalp hair is a strong indication that ODD is a possible diagnosis, although this complex of findings is also common in Hallerman-Streiff syndrome.

Hearing Disorders: Conductive hearing loss has been found in some cases.

Speech Disorders: Articulation impairment is a common manifestation of ODD secondary to small teeth and dental gaps in both the maxillary and mandibular arches. Compensatory articulation secondary to cleft palate and velopharyngeal insufficiency is possible in some cases.

Feeding Disorders: Feeding disorders have not typically been associated with ODD.

Voice Disorders: Voice is normal in ODD.

Resonance Disorders: Hypernasality secondary to cleft palate is a possible finding in some cases.

Language Disorders: Language development is normal.

Other Clinical Features:

  Ocular: short palpebral fissures resulting in small-appearing eyes; microcornea; glaucoma;

  Dental: small teeth; enamel hypoplasia;

  Craniofacial: occasional cleft palate with or without cleft lip; small nose with hypoplastic alar rims; cranial hy-

perostoses; mandibular prognathism; hypotelorism;

  Limbs: contractures of the fifth fingers; syndactyly of the ring finger and little finger and of the third and fourth toes; hypoplasia or aplasia of the middle phalanges, especially of the toes;

  Integument: deficient scalp hair;

  Neurologic: Spastic paraplegia and quadraplegia have been observed in a small number of cases; white matter hyperintensities on magnetic resonance imaging.

Natural History: The structural anomalies associated with ODD are present at birth, except for the dental anomalies that do not become apparent until dental eruption. Developmental milestones are normal and longevity is not affected. In cases with neurologic deficits, the quadraplegia or paraplegia have been progressive.

Treatment Prognosis: Dental anomalies can be treated effectively with bonding or implant procedures. Hypernasality and articulation disorders can be resolved after physical anomalies have been reconstructed. The neurologic disorders seen in some cases must be treated with palliative procedures, such as bracing.

Differential Diagnosis: The eye anomalies combined with the dental malformations in ODD are essentially unique.

OHAHA Syndrome

Also Known As: Ophthalmo-plegia, hypotonia, ataxia, hypo-acusis, and athetosis (OHAHA).

The designation OHAHA syndrome is an acronym probably constructed to provoke a humorous response, a practice that should be viewed with disdain because the joke is at the expense of those who have a serious genetic disease. Individuals with ophthalmoplegia, hypotonia, ataxia, hypoacusis, and athetosis have severe neurologic impairment and fail to develop speech.

Major System(s) Affected: Ocular; central nervous system.

Etiology: Autosomal recessive inheritance. The gene has not been mapped or characterized.

Quick Clues: Affected individuals have hypotonic faciès resulting in an open-mouth posture. Strabismus is also common. Thus, the association of an open-mouth posture with strabismus and progressive sensorineural hearing loss, although not pathognomonic, should raise suspicion of this diagnosis.

Hearing Disorders: Progressive bilateral sensorineural hearing loss with a sudden onset in toddler years or early childhood, resulting in a severe to profound deficiency. Vestibular dysfunction is also present. A total absence of caloric response has been noted.

Speech Disorders: Speech typically does not develop in this syndrome.

Feeding Disorders: Feeding may be impaired by hypotonia. Chewing may be significantly compromised by malocclusion and hypotonia.

Voice Disorders: Wet hoarseness during crying has been observed.

Resonance Disorders: Speech does not develop and, therefore, resonance can not be adequately assessed.

Language Disorders: Severe expressive language impairment. Cognition is reportedly normal.

Other Clinical Features:

Ocular: strabismus; ophthalmoplegia;

Central nervous system: hypotonia; athetoid movements; ataxia; polyneuropathy; imbalance.

Natural History: The onset of the disorder and its major symptoms tend to be first noticed just prior to one year of age, although some cases have been slightly later. The neurologic symptoms show some early progression, but some improved function occurs in childhood. Additional degeneration follows in teen years.

Treatment Prognosis: There are no known treatments at this time.

Differential Diagnosis: Many of the symptoms resemble some of the mitochondrial disorders, such as **Kearns-Sayre syndrome.**

Ohdo Syndrome

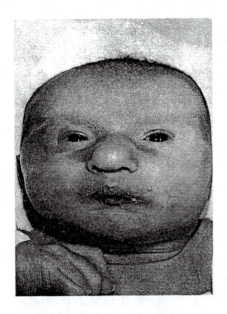

Ohdo syndrome: Note blepharophimosis, microstomia and large nasal tip in Ohdo syndrome.

Also Known As: Ohdo blepharophimosis syndrome; mental retardation, congenital heart disease, blepharophimosis, blepharoptosis, and hypoplastic teeth.

Ohdo syndrome has been described both within families (multiple affected siblings) and in unrelated individuals. All reported cases have had cognitive impairment in combination with distinctive craniofacial findings and conductive hearing loss.

Major System(s) Affected: Craniofacial; cardiac; ocular; central nervous system; genitourinary.

Etiology: Autosomal recessive inheritance. The gene has not been mapped or identified.

Quick Clues: Blepharophimosis in association with mental retardation provides a diagnostic clue in relation to Ohdo syndrome.

Hearing Disorders: Conductive hearing loss is a nearly constant feature. The auricles tend to be small and the external auditory canals narrow.

Speech Disorders: Speech is delayed secondary to cognitive impairment.

Feeding Disorders: Early feeding disorders have not been described.

Voice Disorders: Voice disorders have not been described.

Resonance Disorders: Resonance disorder has not been described.

Language Disorders: Language is impaired secondary to cognitive impairment and potentially complicated by hearing loss.

Other Clinical Features:

> **Craniofacial:** blepharophimosis; small ears; stenotic ear canals; broad nasal root; small teeth;

> **Cardiac:** heart anomalies;

> **Ocular:** amblyopia;

> **Central nervous system:** cognitive impairment;

> **Genitourinary:** cryptorchidism.

Natural History: The anomalies in Ohdo syndrome are congenital and static.

Treatment Prognosis: The prognosis is limited by cognitive development. Conductive hearing loss can be treated effectively and the blepharophimosis can be surgically treated in order to avoid secondary visual impairment.

Differential Diagnosis: Blepharophimosis is found in **Michels syndrome,** but cleft lip and palate are not found in Ohdo syndrome.

Opitz Syndrome

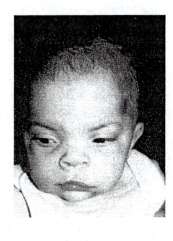

Opitz syndrome: Note hypertelorism.

Also Known As: G syndrome; BBB syndrome; G/BBB syndrome; Opitz-Frias syndrome; hypospadias-dysphagia syndrome; hypertelorism-hypospadias syndrome.

Opitz syndrome has been the focus of some recent attention because of some clinical overlap between it and **velo-cardio-facial syndrome.** The clinical overlap between these two conditions has led some to believe that Opitz syndrome is also caused by a deletion of multiple genes at 22q11.2. However, the condition initially described by Opitz is clearly X-linked and does not resemble **velo-cardio-facial syndrome** at all. Cases with hypertelorism and hypospadias that are deleted at 22q11.2 have **velo-cardio-facial syndrome,** not Opitz syndrome. The problem is not one of genetic heterogeneity, but rather one of diagnostic accuracy.

Major System(s) Affected: Craniofacial; genitourinary; gastrointestinal; central nervous system; cardiac.

Etiology: X-linked recessive inheritance. The gene has been mapped to Xp22 and has been labeled *OSX.*

Quick Clues: Significant and easily recognized hypertelorism in association with a history of hypospadias or laryngeal anomalies should raise the suspicion of the diagnosis. Mothers who are carriers will often have mild hypertelorism, but no other clinical features.

Hearing Disorders: Although not reported or commonly observed in the syndrome, the author has seen several cases of Opitz syndrome with sensorineural hearing loss, including one patient who had a profound impairment. Conductive hearing loss secondary to chronic fluid and middle ear effusion is also common.

Speech Disorders: Speech onset is typically delayed and articulation may be neurologically impaired. Cleft palate with or without cleft lip often results in compensatory articulation patterns secondary to velopharyngeal insufficiency.

Feeding Disorders: Early feeding is almost always impaired with aspiration secondary to laryngotracheoesophageal cleft. Hypotonia also complicates matters and may lead to upper airway obstruction. Esophageal dismotility has been reported, but is a presumptive diagnosis. G-E reflux has also been observed.

Voice Disorders: Hoarse and/or breathy voice are common manifestations of the laryngotracheal clefts associated with Opitz syndrome.

Resonance Disorders: Hypernasality secondary to cleft palate and velopharyngeal insufficiency are common.

Language Disorders: Language is typically delayed and significantly impaired commensurate with cognitive deficiency. Cognitive impairment with mild to moderate mental retardation is a common, but not constant, feature.

Other Clinical Features:

> **Craniofacial:** hypertelorism; cleft palate with or without cleft lip; ankyloglossia;

> **Genitourinary:** hypospadias; small male genitalia; bifid scrotum; renal or ureteral anomalies;

> **Gastrointestinal:** laryngotracheoesophageal cleft; occasional imperforate anus; umbilical hernia;

> **Central nervous system:** cognitive impairment; agenesis of the corpus callosum;

Cardiac: coarctation of the aorta; atrial septal defect.

Natural History: The initial presentation of the syndrome is a weak cry and aspiration during feeding secondary to the laryngeal cleft. Hypotonia and developmental delay become apparent, when present, in infancy. The genital hypoplasia and anomalies are also present at birth. Development is globally delayed in those cases with cognitive deficiency.

Treatment Prognosis: The prognosis is variable, depending on the presence of cognitive impairment and central nervous system anomalies. Reconstruction of the laryngeal cleft becomes necessary, but tracheotomy is obviously necessary in many cases until reconstruction has been complete.

Differential Diagnosis: Velo-cardio-facial syndrome has many of the same phenotypic features as Opitz syndrome, including hypospadias, occasional mild hypertelorism, cleft palate, developmental delay, hoarse voice (secondary to paresis or laryngeal web), hypotonia, and congenital heart anomalies. However, the appearance of the ears, nose, and digits is different from that seen in Opitz syndrome.

Oral-Facial-Digital Syndrome

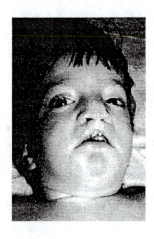 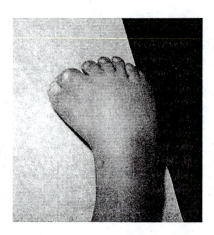

Oral-facial-digital syndromes: Note the cleft lip and palate associated with preaxial and postaxial polydactyly of the foot.

Also Known As: OFD.

The oral-facial-digital syndromes are a group of eight separate disorders, each with a different genetic cause, but grouped together under the nosologic category of OFD because of the similarities in phenotypic expression, particularly in relation to the lobulated tongue and multiple oral frenula. For the sake of convenience, all the disorders are listed under this single entry with each subtype's genotype and phenotype listed separately, except for

Mohr syndrome, which is listed separately under that commonly used heading.

Major System(s) Affected: Craniofacial/oral (all subtypes); limbs (all subtypes); integument (OFD1), central nervous system (all subtypes except OFD5), renal (OFD7).

Etiology: OFD1 and OFD8 are both X-linked recessive. OFD3, OFD4, OFD5, and OFD6 are all autosomal recessive. OFD7 is probably autosomal dominant. OFD1 has been mapped to Xp22.3-p22.2. The other subtypes have not been mapped.

Quick Clues: The association of polydactyly with abnormal oral findings such as cleft lip, midline notching of the lip, abnormal oral frenulae, or lobulation of the tongue should point strongly to one of the OFD syndromes as a diagnosis.

Hearing Disorders: Conductive hearing loss has been demonstrated and observed in OFD1 and OFD4.

Speech Disorders: All the oral-facial digital syndromes are marked by significant speech delay. OFD1 is distinguished by eventual dysarthria. All the oral-facial digital syndromes have articulatory impairment related to abnormal tongue anatomy and the presence of hyperplastic oral frenulae.

Feeding Disorders: Early failure-to-thrive is common in all types of OFD except OFD5 secondary to cognitive impairment and central nervous system malformations. A substantial number of patients with OFD do not survive infancy.

Voice Disorders: Voice disorders have not been observed in the oral-facial digital syndromes.

Resonance Disorders: Hypernasality secondary to cleft palate may occur in OFD1, OFD4, and OFD6.

Language Disorders: Language impairment, often severe, is common in OFD1, OFD2, OFD3, OFD4, OFD6, OFD7, and OFD8. In the most severe cases, there is essentially no functional language development.

Other Clinical Features:

Craniofacial/oral: midline cleft or notch of the upper lip (OFD1, OFD5, OFD7); cleft lip with or without cleft palate (OFD4, OFD6, OFD8); lobulated tongue, hyperplastic oral frenulae;

Limbs: polydactyly;

Integument: multiple milia along the ears (OFD1);

Central nervous system: absence of the corpus callosum; porencephaly; cognitive impairment (all subtypes except OFD5);

Renal: kidney dysfunction (OFD7).

Natural History: All anomalies are present at birth. With the exception of OFD5, there is a high probability of marked delay of psychomotor development.

Treatment Prognosis: Prognosis is dependent on the degree of cognitive impairment. The digital and tongue anomalies can be managed surgically.

Differential Diagnosis: The challenge with the oral-facial-digital syndromes is distinguishing each one from the other, in large part because of the need to provide appropriate genetic counseling.

Otopalatodigital Syndrome, Type 1

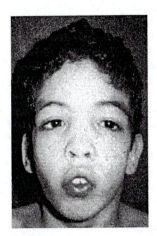
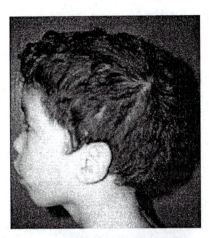

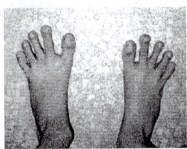
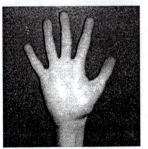

Otopalatodigital syndrome type 1: Note the mild hypertelorism, downslanting palpebral fissures, and micrognathia (top row). The toes show shortened halluces and thickened finger pads with curved digits (bottom row).

Also Known As: OPD1.

Otopalatodigital syndrome is a syndrome of cleft palate, micrognathia, and digital anomalies that also has the Robin sequence as an associated finding. The digit anomalies are distinctive. Although there are nosologically two forms of otopalatodigital syndrome, and both are X-linked, there is little similarity between the two conditions in that the facial and digital anomalies are distinctively different. Female heterozygotes tend to show minor manifestations of the gene, including minor digital anomalies.

Major System(s) Affected: Craniofacial; limbs; auditory; central nervous system; dental, growth.

Etiology: X-linked recessive inheritance. The gene has been mapped to Xq28.

Quick Clues: The anomalies of the fingers are distinctive (thickened finger pads and clinodactyly), and when associated with some limitation of bend at the elbow, OPD1 should be considered as a diagnosis.

Hearing Disorders: Conductive hearing loss is common and is re-lated to both ossicular anomalies and chronic middle ear effusion.

Speech Disorders: Speech is typically delayed, usually mildly. Eventually speech is marked by articulation impairment related to malocclusion, including anterior skeletal open-bite. Tongue-backing is also common because of micrognathia and occasional ankyloglossia. Compensatory articulation disorders secondary to cleft palate and velopharyngeal insufficiency are common.

Feeding Disorders: Early failure-to-thrive is common and is almost always related to airway obstruction, which is prompted by the combination of micrognathia, an acute cranial base angle, and hypotonia. Resolution of the airway compromise will resolve the feeding problems.

Voice Disorders: Voice is typically normal.

Resonance Disorders: Cleft palate is a very common finding in the syndrome so that hypernasal speech is common.

Language Disorders: Language delay is a nearly constant finding with expressive language being somewhat more severely impaired than receptive. The degree of language involvement may be more significant than cognitive impairment would predict. Many cases have low normal intelligence, and most are borderline or have mild mental retardation.

Other Clinical Features:

> **Craniofacial:** micrognathia; "pugilistic facies" with prominent brow and frontal bossing; broad nasal root; hypertelorism; downslanting eyes; downslanting oral commissures; acute cranial base angle;

> **Limbs:** short halluces; widely spaced toes; clinodactyly; thick finger and toe pads; radial head dislocation; broad thumbs; short fingernails;

> **Skeletal:** osteochondrodysplasia; scoliosis; pectus excavatum secondary to airway obstruction;

> **Auditory:** conductive hearing loss;

> **Central nervous system:** cognitive impairment;

> **Dental:** hypodontia;

> **Growth:** small stature.

Natural History: The digital anomalies may be difficult to recognize at birth and in infancy, as are the facial anomalies. The first signs of the syndrome may be cleft palate and failure-to-thrive. With age, the digital anomalies become more obvious and are very distinctive in appearance.

Treatment Prognosis: The prognosis is typically good with speech and language disorders being amenable to therapy. Hearing disorders require amplification.

Differential Diagnosis: Digital, clefting, and micrognathia are common in **otopalatodigital syndrome, type 2** (OPD2), and **Nager syndrome,** but the distinctive appearance of the toes and fingers in OPD1 leaves little room for confusion.

Otopalatodigital Syndrome, Type 2

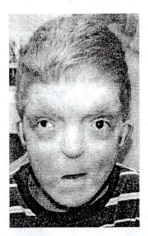

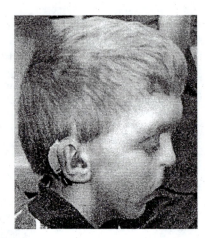

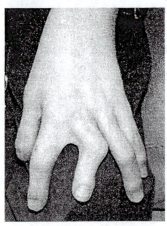

Otopalatodigital syndrome type 2: Note the hypertelorism and micrognathia associated with syndactyly and contractures.

Also Known As: OPD2; cranio-orodigital syndrome.

OPD2 is a rare syndrome that has been recognized infrequently and may be under-reported or diagnosed as another entity. The phenotype is more severe than **OPD1** and actually does not resemble it particularly, except for the groupings of anomaly types. Although both syndromes have limb anomalies, the anomalies are not similar.

Major System(s) Affected: Craniofacial; limbs; skeletal; genitourinary; abdominal; central nervous system.

Etiology: X-linked recessive.

Quick Clues: The severe clinodactyly and camptodactyly of OPD2 are distinctive and are always accompanied by significant craniofacial manifestations. The microstomia is a strong diagnostic clue.

Hearing Disorders: Conductive hearing loss secondary to ossicular malformations and fusions have been observed.

Speech Disorders: Speech is marked by severe articulation impairment including retraction of all articulation in the posterior portion of the oral cavity, because the entire oropharyngeal cavity is extremely small, including the mouth. The tongue is small, as is the mandible. Lingual protrusion is difficult and there may be significant ankyloglossia. Articulation is often in the floor of the mouth, with poor tongue movement within the maxillary arch.

Feeding Disorders: Early failure-to-thrive and feeding disorders are common secondary to upper airway obstruction. There is very limited oral opening and glossoptosis. Aggressive management of the airway problems is recommended prior to alternative approaches to feeding.

Voice Disorders: Voice is normal.

Resonance Disorders: Resonance is a mix of hypernasality (secondary to cleft palate) and muffled oral resonance (secondary to a small oropharynx and oral cavity). Although velopharyngeal insufficiency is common, the airway below the velopharyngeal valve is so limited in size, even in rest position, that the disordered resonance balance may be more severely impaired in the oral cavity than in the nasal cavity.

Language Disorders: Language development is often normal, but some cases have had hydrocephalus and secondary effects on the central nervous system. Cognitive impairment has also been observed in some cases. Language impairment is commensurate to the degree of cognitive involvement.

Other Clinical Features:

Craniofacial: maxillary and mandibular hypoplasia; small mouth; cleft palate; downturned oral commissures; hypertelorism; downslanting eyes; broad, high forehead;

Limbs: syndactyly; contractures; clinodactyly; bowing of the limbs; limitation of joint extension; absent fibula;

Skeletal: narrow chest;

Genitourinary: hypospadias; hydronephrosis; hydroureter;

Abdominal: omphalocele;

Central nervous system: hydrocephalus; occasional cognitive impairment.

Natural History: All anomalies are present at birth. Hydrocephalus may be noticed in infancy secondary to abnormal head shape and head circumference. Airway obstruction and failure-to-thrive are common in infancy.

Treatment Prognosis: The prognosis is, in part, dependent on the presence or absence of central nervous system involvement. Skeletal structures can be managed surgically in many cases, including the hypoplasia of the mandible. Mandibular distraction may have a place in the management of the facial skeleton.

Differential Diagnosis: OPD1 has craniofacial and digital anomalies, but without the broader spectrum of skeletal malformations. The craniofacial features in OPD2 are somewhat reminiscent of syndromes of craniosynostosis.

Pendred Syndrome

Also Known As: Deafness with goiter; goiter-deafness syndrome.

Pendred syndrome is an autosomal recessive syndrome of hearing loss with accompanying thyroid enlargement beginning in childhood. There is variable expression of the clinical features of the syndrome, including the hearing loss and cochlear anomaly. However, the association of goiter and hearing loss is a distinctive one.

Major System(s) Affected: Endocrine; central nervous system.

Etiology: Autosomal recessive inheritance. The gene has been mapped to 7q31.

Quick Clues: An enlarged thyroid gland with thickening around the neck in association with sensorineural hearing loss is a strong indication of Pendred syndrome.

Hearing Disorders: Hearing loss may be congenital or have its onset in childhood. The hearing loss is bilateral and may be progressive, ranging from moderate to profound. Vestibular dysfunction may also be found. A Mondini type anomaly of the cochlea has been observed on multiple occasions in individuals with Pendred syndrome. Vestibular function is depressed in less than half of affected individuals.

Speech Disorders: Speech development is typically normal in early childhood, unless the hearing loss is congenital and severe.

Feeding Disorders: There are no feeding disorders in childhood, but if the goiter becomes extremely large, subsequent sensations of globus and airway constriction are possible.

Voice Disorders: Hoarseness may be caused by a severe goiter.

Resonance Disorders: Resonance is normal.

Language Disorders: Language development is normal unless hearing loss is congenital and severe.

P

Other Clinical Features:

> **Endocrine:** euthyroidism; goiter; occasional thyroid carcinoma;
>
> **Central nervous system:** occasional cognitive impairment.

Natural History: Hearing loss is occasionally congenital, but more often has an onset in early childhood and then may become progressively worse. Similarly, the onset of thyroid enlargement is also found in childhood with progressive worsening.

Treatment Prognosis: Palliative treatment for thyroid dysfunction is possible and effective. Hearing loss may be treated effectively with amplification.

Differential Diagnosis: Hypothyroidism is a common feature of **velo-cardio-facial syndrome,** which also includes sensorineural hearing loss and cognitive impairment as clinical features.

Pfeiffer Syndrome

Pfeiffer syndrome is one of the well-recognized syndromes of craniosynostosis. Three subtypes of the disorder are now recognized. Pfeiffer syndrome, type 1 is the classically described phenotype of craniosynostosis and broad thumbs. In type 2, the disorder is characterized by cloverleaf skull, or kleeblattschädel, and limitation of movement at the elbows. Pfeiffer syndrome, type 3 has abnormalities of the gut and viscera in association with craniosynostosis and severe shortening of the anterior cranial base. Types 2 and 3 are fatal in infancy.

Major System(s) Affected: Craniofacial; limbs, central nervous system.

Etiology: Autosomal dominant inheritance. The gene has been mapped to two different loci. One mutation occurs in fibroblast growth factor receptor 2 (*FGFR2*), mapped to 10q26. The other mutation is in fibroblast growth factor receptor 1 (*FGFR1*), mapped to 8p11.2-p11.1. Type 2 and type 3 forms of the disorder have more severe craniofacial anomalies and appear to be incompatible with long term survival. Specifically, the skull in types 2 and 3 presents with the kleeblättschadel anomaly (clover leaf skull), with severe shortening of the anterior skull base. Unlike type 2, type 3 Pfeiffer syndrome has anomalies of the gut, including prune belly and bowel malformations. As types 2 and 3 are rarely encountered clinically, because of early demise, Pfeiffer syndrome type 1 will be described in this section.

Quick Clues: The craniofacial manifestations of the syndromes associated with 10q26 mutations are all relatively similar (**Crouzon, Apert,** and Pfeiffer syndromes) and easily recognized. Therefore, narrowing down the diagnosis may often be relegated to examination of the limbs. Although broad thumbs and halluces are common manifestations of Pfeiffer syndrome and can be used as inclusive features for the diagnosis, the presence of multidigit syndactyly or normal limbs can be exlusive for the diagnosis.

Hearing Disorders: Conductive hearing loss is common, often reaching the moderate to severe range. Ossicular fusions have been found.

Speech Disorders: Articulation is impaired secondary to a Class III malocclusion caused by maxillary hypoplasia. The tongue tends to articulate in the mandibular arch with limited maxillary contact. All anterior sounds are distorted or substitutions made. These errors are obligatory and are related to the severity of the malocclusion. Anterior skeletal open-bite is common and results in lingual protrusion. Speech onset is delayed in a small percentage of cases secondary to neurologic complications, such as hydrocephalus.

Feeding Disorders: Early feeding is often impaired secondary to airway compromise. Airway obstruction has multiple sources, including choanal atresia or stenosis, pharyngeal obstruction secondary to maxillary hypoplasia and the palate hanging deeply into the oropharynx, and in some cases, rigidity of the trachea caused by a solid cartilaginous tube rather than the normal ring-like structure.

Voice Disorders: Hoarse voice is common, especially in cases with tracheal anomalies.

Resonance Disorders: Hyponasality is common secondary to choanal stenosis or atresia, and also because of maxillary hypoplasia that decreases the total volume of the nasopharyngeal airway. Oral resonance may also be impaired, with a muffled resonance caused by reduced maxillary volume and a reduction in oral cavity size.

Language Disorders: Language development is typically normal except in the small percentage of cases with neurological complications.

Other Clinical Features:

> **Craniofacial:** craniosynostosis of multiple sutures; acrocephaly; increased intracranial pressure; maxillary hypoplasia; shallow orbits; hypertelorism; downslanting palpebral fissures; choanal stenosis or atresia; soft tissue hypertrophy of the palatal shelves (pseudocleft); exophthalmos; Class III malocclusion;

Limbs: broad thumbs and halluces; radially deviated thumbs; mild soft tissue syndactyly; brachydactyly; occasional polysyndactyly of the thumbs or halluces;

Central nervous system: occasional hydrocephalus; occasional Arnold-Chiari anomaly.

Natural History: At birth, many babies with Pfeiffer syndrome have relatively normal facial appearance. Anthropometric measurement may yield evidence of hypertelorism. The anterior fontanel is often patent and remains that way through the first year of life. However, maxillary hypoplasia and acrocephaly become evident with growth. Increased intracranial pressure may also develop. With normal mandibular growth throughout childhood and maxillary hypoplasia, relative prognathism becomes evident before school age.

Treatment Prognosis: Craniofacial reconstruction can prevent the increase in intracranial pressure from becoming severe. Choanal stenosis or atresia cannot be permanently resolved with surgery because ossification of the craniofacial skeleton is progressive and continues throughout life. Airway obstruction may be life-threatening in many cases and tracheotomy is often necessary. Craniofacial reconstruction may be performed for the midfacial hypoplasia.

Differential Diagnosis: The craniofacial anomalies in Pfeiffer syndrome are similar to those seen in **Crouzon syndrome, Jackson-Weiss syndrome,** and **Apert syndrome.** The syndromes can be differentiated based on the limb anomalies. **Sathre-Chotzen syndrome** has similar soft tissue syndactyly of the hands, but the craniofacial anomalies are different from those found in Pfeiffer syndrome.

P

Pontobulbar Palsy with Sensorineural Hearing Loss

Also Known As: Brown-Vialetto-van Laere syndrome; progressive bulbar palsy with perceptive deafness.

This syndrome of degenerative neurological complications is important to identify early because management of feeding disorders can be beneficial for avoiding potentially fatal complications of aspiration. Essentially all the earliest manifestations of the disorder are communicative in nature, and audiologists and speech-language pathologists may often be the first professionals to come in contact with affected individuals.

Major System(s) Affected: Auditory; central nervous system.

Etiology: Autosomal recessive, autosomal dominant, and X-linked inheritance have all been hypothesized based on pedigree analysis of a number of families with multiple affected individuals. It is unclear if this represents etiologic heterogeneity versus a number of close phenocopies caused by different genes.

Quick Clues: Lower cranial nerve palsies associated with a rapid degeneration of hearing are a strong indication of pontobulbar palsy.

Hearing Disorders: In most cases, the first clinical expression of the syndrome is sensorineural hearing loss. Hearing loss usually appears in childhood in the primary school years, although some cases have demonstrated an early onset, while others have not had clinical manifestations until late teen years.

Speech Disorders: Speech onset and early development is normal. After the onset of the disease, weak oral consonant production follows. The tongue develops fasciculations followed by dysarthria.

Feeding Disorders: Dysphagia with aspiration and true bulbar-based disorders of swallowing eventually develop as the disease progresses. Diminished pharyngeal and laryngeal sensation and vocal cord paralysis are common in the end-stages of the disorder.

Voice Disorders: Initially, voice is normal. After the onset of the disorder, voice is initially hoarse, followed by breathiness, and eventually dysphonia or aphonia related to vocal cord paresis.

Resonance Disorders: An early manifestation of the disorder is the onset of hypernasal speech and nasal air emission.

Language Disorders: Language development is normal.

Other Clinical Features:

    Auditory: Sensorineural hearing loss with occasionally very rapid progression;

    Central nervous system: lower cranial nerve palsies; lower motor neuron dysfunction; hypoactive reflexes; muscle wasting.

Natural History: The first noticeable symptom is usually hearing loss, although in some cases, upper eyelid ptosis may appear earlier. Hearing loss is followed by speech and resonance disorders, and then swallowing and respiratory complications. The disorder may have either very rapid or slow progression. In cases with rapid progression, early demise may occur secondary to respiratory complications, including diaphragmatic paresis, aspiration, and pulmonary insufficiency.

Treatment Prognosis: In cases with milder progression, alternative strategies for feeding may be very helpful in avoiding dangerous complications of bulbar palsy. Hypernasality will respond to prosthetic management, specifically obturation. Surgery is contraindicated because the disease is progressive.

Differential Diagnosis: There are a number of other rare disorders with similar progressive symptoms, including Fazio-Londe disease.

P

Refsum Syndrome

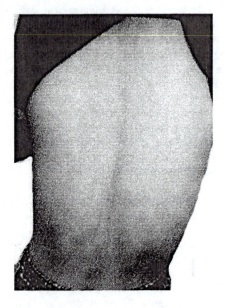

Refsum syndrome: Ichthyosis of the skin on the back in Refsum syndrome.

Also Known As: Refsum disease; heredopathia atactica polyneuritiformis; phytanic acid oxidase deficiency.

First delineated in 1946, this is one of the syndromes of deafness that has the association of retinitis pigmentosa with sensorineural hearing loss. Unlike **Usher syndrome,** Refsum syndrome has progressive neurologic abnormalities that are associated with progressive build-up of phytanic acid. Typically of relatively late onset (second or third decade of life), there is also an infantile onset form that is a different clinical entity from the syndrome initially delineated.

Major System(s) Affected: Auditory; metabolic; ocular; neurologic; musculoskeletal; integument; cardiac.

Etiology: Autosomal recessive inheritance. A mutation in the

PAHX gene at 10pter-p11.2 has been identified.

Quick Clues: Ichthyosis accompanied by peripheral neurologic degeneration is a strong indicator of Refsum syndrome.

Hearing Disorders: Sensorineural hearing loss is of relatively late onset, usually in late teen years or slightly after. The onset of the hearing loss may be unilateral. The hearing loss is progressive and gradually reaches severe to profound levels over a period of 10 or more years. Although the initial onset may be asymmetric, over time the impairment becomes symmetric with increasing severity. High frequencies are more severely affected. Vestibular function is typically normal.

Speech Disorders: Speech develops normally because the hearing loss does not become expressed until later in life. The majority of neurologic symptoms begin in the limbs and do not affect the speech mechanism until much later, if at all. On occasion, some dysarthria may occur.

Feeding Disorders: Feeding is normal in early life and is rarely affected later in life.

Voice Disorders: Voice is normal, but in the latest stages of the disorder may become weak or tremulous.

Resonance Disorders: Resonance is normal.

Language Disorders: Language development is normal.

Other Clinical Features:

> **Metabolic:** Abnormal fatty acid metabolism; phytanic acid oxidase deficiency and accumulation of phytanic acid in multiple tissues;
>
> **Ocular:** retinitis pigmentosa; ptosis; miosis;
>
> **Neurologic:** polyneuritis; ataxia; anosmia;
>
> **Musculoskeletal:** epiphyseal dysplasia;
>
> **Integument:** ichthyosis;
>
> **Cardiac:** arrhythmias; congestive heart failure.

Natural History: Affected individuals do not show significant manifestations of the syndrome in childhood. The first noticeable onset may be in late teen years with the development of night blindness. The progression is then slow with the onset of polyneuritis, peripheral wasting, ichthyosis, and eventually more severe peripheral neurologic findings, including ataxia and eventual paralysis in some cases. Cardiac arrhythmias may be life threatening if not treated.

Treatment Prognosis: The prognosis is typically good until the late stages of the disease which may be in late middle or old age.

Differential Diagnosis: The association of hearing loss and retinitis pigmentosa is most commonly seen in **Usher syndrome.** Most forms of **Usher syndrome** do not have the neurologic symptoms of Refsum (except for type IA) and the metabolic symptoms of Refsum syndrome are unique.

Rubella Embryopathy

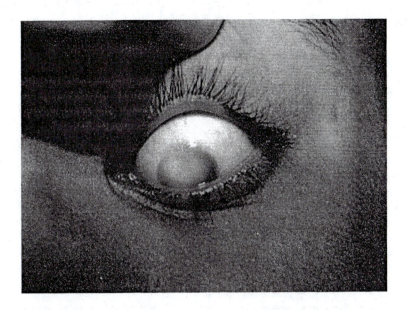

Rubella embryopathy: Congenital cataract in rubella embryopathy.

Also Known As: Fetal rubella syndrome.

Viral infections may have teratogenic influences if the virus infects the developing embryo. The expression of the syndrome is dependent on the timing of the infection. An expansive phenotype is present when the infection is contracted within the first trimester.

When the infection occurs during the second trimester, the major effect is typically short stature.

Major System(s) Affected: Ocular; central nervous system; cardiac; hematologic; internal organs; genitourinary; endocrine; skeletal.

Etiology: Rubella infection (teratogenic).

Quick Clues: The presence of congenital cataracts in association with developmental impairment and sensorineural hearing loss is indicative of rubella embryopathy. Historical information is obviously of primary importance.

Hearing Disorders: Bilateral congenital sensorineural hearing loss, typically profound, is the norm.

Speech Disorders: In the most severe cases, speech does not develop because of severe mental retardation. In milder cases, speech is affected by congenital deafness or profound hearing loss.

Feeding Disorders: In the most severe cases, severe neurological symptoms and hypotonia result in early failure-to-thrive.

Voice Disorders: Specific voice impairments have not been noted.

Resonance Disorders: Resonance may be impaired secondary to severe neurologic impairment in the most severe cases.

Language Disorders: In the most severe cases, expressive language may not develop, and receptive language may be severely impaired. In milder cases, language skills may be within the normal range.

Other Clinical Features:

Ocular: congenital cataracts; corneal opacification; congenital glaucoma; microphthalmia; strabismus;

Central nervous system: primary microcephaly; cognitive impairment;

Cardiac: ventriculoseptal defect; atrial septal defect; myocardial disease; pulmonary atresia or stenosis;

Hematologic: thrombocytopenia; anemia;

Viscera: hepatosplenomegaly; jaundice;

Genitourinary: hypospadias; renal anomalies; cryptorchidism;

Endocrine: diabetes mellitus; short stature; pituitary deficiency;

Skeletal: bone lesions.

Natural History: The anomalies associated with fetal rubella embryopathy are all present at birth and do not progress.

Treatment Prognosis: The prognosis for treatment is dependent on the severity of central nervous system impairment, when present. In the most severe cases, the prognosis for improvement and response to treatment is extremely poor.

Differential Diagnosis: Congenital cataracts are also caused by the teratogenic effects of **cytomegalovirus.** Corneal opacification is found in **Harboyan syndrome,** but without the central nervous system impairment seen in rubella embryopathy.

R

Rubinstein-Taybi Syndrome

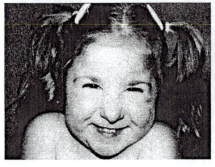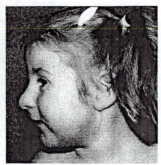

Rubinstein-Taybi syndrome

Also Known As: Rubinstein syndrome; broad thumb-hallux syndrome.

Rubinstein-Taybi syndrome is a relatively common syndrome of mental retardation among individuals that are institutionalized. The population frequency is low, perhaps 1:300,000. The combination of distinctive craniofacial, developmental, heart, and limb anomalies is easily recognized.

Major System(s) Affected: Central nervous system; craniofacial; growth; limbs; cardiac; integument; ocular; musculoskeletal; gastrointestinal; genitourinary.

Etiology: Autosomal dominant inheritance. The gene has been mapped to 16p13.3 and the gene has been labeled *CBP* for CREB Binding Protein, and mutations of this gene, including deletions, have been identified. The *CBP* gene acts to bind two proteins together and this binding process eventually activates other genes. Mutations in *CBP* prevent the binding, and thus the activation, of other genes.

Quick Clues: The beak-shaped nose, downslanting eyes, downslanting oral commissures, and long upcurled eyelashes make a distinctive complex of facial findings.

Hearing Disorders: Conductive hearing loss is found in nearly a quarter of individuals with Rubinstein-Taybi syndrome.

Speech Disorders: A high percentage of individuals with Rubinstein-Taybi syndrome do not develop speech. Those who do develop speech usually display severe impairment of articulation, rhythm, and rate, often with significant dysarthria. Children are often labeled as dyspraxic. Speech is often unintelligible.

Feeding Disorders: Early failure-to-thrive is common and is precipitated by hypotonia, congenital heart anomalies, micrognathia, laryngomalacia, and airway obstruction. Chronic constipation also contributes to abdominal discomfort that decreases desire to feed.

Voice Disorders: Hoarseness and high pitch have been observed in many cases.

Resonance Disorders: Hypernasal resonance has been observed as a component of dysarthric speech related to hypotonia. However, even when present, hypernasality has not been a major contributor to unintelligibility, as has the speech production disorder.

Language Disorders: Language impairment is a constant, and expressive language is always more severely impaired than receptive language. Many individuals with Rubinstein-Taybi syndrome have good language comprehension but essentially no functional speech.

Other Clinical Features:

> **Central nervous system:** mental retardation, typically moderate, with the majority of IQs below 50; seizures; hyperactive deep tendon reflexes; hypoplasia or absence of the corpus callosum; hypotonia; psychiatric illness;

> **Craniofacial:** microcephaly; large anterior fontanel; mild hypertelorism; downslanting eyes; micrognathia; mild facial asymmetry; beak-shaped nose; downslanting oral commissures; long eyelashes;

> **Growth:** short stature;

> **Limbs:** broad thumbs and halluces; hyperextensible joints; radially deviated thumbs; broad distal phalanges on all digits;

> **Cardiac:** ventricular and atrial septal defects; patent

R

ductus arteriosus; coarctation of the aorta; conduction abnormalities; pulmonary stenosis; mitral valve insufficiency; cardiomyopathy; cor pulmonale;

Integument: hirsutism; capillary hemangiomas; supernumerary nipples; keloid formation;

Ocular: strabismus; nasolacrimal duct obstruction; ptosis; ocular coloboma; cataracts; glaucoma;

Musculoskeletal: spina bifida occulta; scoliosis; kyphosis; frequent fractures; abnormal femoral epiphyses; short sternum;

Gastrointestinal: constipation, aganglionic megacolon;

Genitourinary: renal hypoplasia/aplasia; cryptorchidism.

Natural History: The facial manifestations of Rubinstein-Taybi syndrome are not always obvious at birth or in infancy, and broadening of the thumbs and halluces is difficult to appreciate when the hands and feet are very small. Therefore, many cases of Rubinstein-Taybi syndrome are diagnosed relatively

late in life, often during childhood or at school age. One of the earliest presentations, if heart anomalies are not present, is failure-to-thrive and chronic constipation, followed by developmental delay. The onset of speech is usually severely delayed. In many individuals with Rubinstein-Taybi syndrome who do develop speech, the onset of first words may not occur until three or four years of age. In many cases, speech consists of a small sample of single words. In those with more speech development, speech is often unintelligible. As adolescence approaches, maladaptive behaviors become more common and psychiatric illness involving mood and temperament becomes evident in many cases.

Treatment Prognosis: The prognosis for normal speech development is typically poor. In many cases, because receptive language is more intact, the potential for expressive language might appear good. However, if the onset of significant speech does not occur by school age, the prognosis for considerable speech development is typically poor.

Differential Diagnosis: Broad thumbs and halluces, as well as beaked nose and hypertelorism, are common findings in **Pfeiffer syndrome.** However, the presence of heart anomalies would negate the diagnosis of **Pfeiffer.** Because of the unusual facial appearance in Rubinstein-Taybi syndrome, the diagnosis of **de Lange syndrome** has been made incorrectly in some cases. Coarctation of the aorta, ASD, VSD, developmental delay, severe speech delay, psychiatric illness, and unusual facial appearance are also found in **velo-cardio-facial syndrome,** but there is little similarity in the facial phenotype with advancing age.

Saethre-Chotzen Syndrome

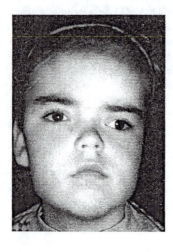

Saethre-Chotzen syndrome: Note orbital and facial asymmetry.

Also Known As: Acrocephalosyndactyly, type III.

Saethre-Chotzen syndrome is one of the least recognized and diagnosed syndromes of craniosynostosis. There is little resemblance between Saethre-Chotzen and **Crouzon, Apert,** or **Pfeiffer syndromes,** even though Saethre-Chotzen syndrome has been labeled as one of the acrocephalosyndactyly disorders.

Major System(s) Affected:
Craniofacial; limbs; ocular; cardiac; central nervous system.

Etiology: Autosomal dominant inheritance. The gene has been mapped to 7p21 and has been identified as the *TWIST* transcription factor gene.

Quick Clues: Although the features of Saethre-Chotzen syndrome are often mild and subtle, the association of either brachycephaly or acrocephaly with asymmetry of the cranium should raise an index of suspicion.

Hearing Disorders: Conductive hearing loss is relatively common, but not a constant finding. In some cases, the hearing loss is unilateral and is typically mild to moderate.

Speech Disorders: In the small percentage of cases with cognitive impairment, there may be delayed onset of speech development. Speech production is otherwise typically normal.

Feeding Disorders: Feeding disorders have not been reported or observed.

Voice Disorders: Voice production is normal.

Resonance Disorders: Nasal resonance disorders of both types have been observed, including hypernasality secondary to cleft palate and velopharyngeal insufficiency, and hyponasality secondary to reduced diameter of the nasopharynx.

Language Disorders: Language is impaired in a small percentage of cases, specifically those that have cognitive impairment.

Other Clinical Features:

Craniofacial: craniosynostosis; craniofacial asymmetry; brachycephaly; acrocephaly; cleft palate;

Limbs: lack of extension at elbows and knees; mild soft tissue syndactyly;

Ocular: strabismus;

Cardiac: occasional congenital heart anomalies;

Central nervous system: occasional cognitive impairment.

Natural History: In many instances, the craniosynostosis is evident at birth and may appear to be severe, but cranial growth and shape often improve with age. Development is typically normal.

Treatment Prognosis: The prognosis is typically good and reconstructive surgery may be effective in treating craniofacial and limb anomalies.

Differential Diagnosis: Saethre-Chotzen syndrome is not typically misdiagnosed as one of the other syndromes of craniosynostosis, but the clinical findings are more typically attributed to simple isolated craniosynostosis or plagiocephaly.

Sanfilippo Syndrome

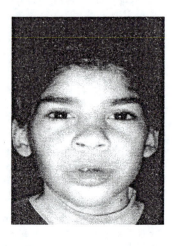

Sanfilippo syndrome: Coarse facial appearance in Sanfilippo syndrome.

Also Known As: Mucopolysaccharidosis type III, with subtypes Mucopolysaccharidosis type IIIA, IIIB, IIIC, and IIID, or as Sanfilippo A, B, C, or D. The difference between the four subtypes is the gene causing the phenotype and the specific enzyme deficiency.

Sanfilippo syndrome is another of the lysosomal storage diseases known as the mucopolysaccharidoses. Several variants of Sanfilippo syndrome have been delineated, each caused by a different gene, but with similar phenotypes. Some estimates for the birth frequency of Sanfilippo syndrome are as high as 1:24,000.

Major System(s) Affected: Growth; craniofacial; central nervous system; musculoskeletal; integument; hepatic.

Etiology: All four subtypes are autosomal recessive disorders. The gene for Sanfilippo A causes a deficiency of heparan N-sulfatase and has been mapped to 17q25.3. The gene for Sanfilippo B has been mapped to 17q21, Sanfilippo C to chromosome 14, and Sanfilippo D to 12q14.

Quick Clues: The presence of aggressive and maladaptive behavior in association with progressive coarsening of the facial appearance is a strong diagnostic clue.

Hearing Disorders: Conductive hearing loss secondary to chronic and severe middle ear effusion is common and progressive. Onset is typically at about school age.

Speech Disorders: Early speech milestones are typically normal, but in early childhood, developmental delay becomes apparent. Any speech that is attained in childhood is eventually lost.

Feeding Disorders: Early feeding is normal, but with advancing expression of the disorder, chronic airway difficulty and deteriorating neurologic function result in difficult feeding. Eventual loss of bulbar function makes normal oral feeding impossible.

Voice Disorders: Voice becomes hoarse with the progression of the disorder. There may be a behavioral component because children become aggressive and many have temper tantrums with screaming.

Resonance Disorders: Resonance eventually becomes hyponasal as chronic mucous fills the nasal cavity and mucous membranes become boggy. There is eventual loss of bulbar function.

Language Disorders: Early language milestones are normal, but delay becomes evident in childhood and deterioration follows.

Other Clinical Features:

Growth: Short stature, typically mild;

Craniofacial: thick calvarial bones; mildly coarse face; macrocephaly;

Central nervous system: eventual mental retardation with progressive deterioration; hyperactivity; aggressiveness; ADD/ADHD; frequent and severe temper tantrums; destructive behavior;

Musculoskeletal: anomalous vertebrae; stiffening of the joints;

Integument: hirsutism;

Hepatic: mild liver enlargement.

Natural History: The onset of the disorder is typically apparent early in the toddler stage as developmental milestones begin to lag behind. An early sign is overactive and aggressive behavior, which is usually apparent before any significant coarsening of the facies. There is often severe sleep disturbance, including both restlessness and eventually obstructive sleep apnea. Eventually, motor control becomes severely impaired. There is progressive ataxia, dementia, seizures; tremors, and eventual bulbar dysfunction that can prevent normal feeding. Most affected individuals do not survive beyond 20 years of age.

Treatment Prognosis: Extremely poor.

Differential Diagnosis: The phenotype and progressive nature of the disorder is similar to other lysosomal storage diseases and metabolic disorders. There are definitive molecular tests that can confirm the diagnosis of Sanfilippo syndrome (for all types).

Seitelberger Syndrome

Also Known As: Infantile neuroaxonal dystrophy; Seitelberger disease.

Seitelberger syndrome is a degenerative neurological disorder of infancy that is probably one of the most common disorders of its type. The disorder has a rapid progressive course that ultimately results in the child's demise, with feeding, speech, and hearing disorders all common manifestations of the syndrome.

Major System(s) Affected: Central nervous system; ocular; endocrine; circulation.

Etiology: Autosomal recessive inheritance. The gene has not been mapped or identified.

Quick Clues: The association of nystagmus and the absence of tearing is a distinctive combination in Seitelberger syndrome.

Hearing Disorders: Toward the end of the progression of the syndrome, sensorineural hearing loss occurs. The hearing loss is difficult to detect because it is accompanied by severe neurologic degeneration and dementia.

Speech Disorders: Initial speech milestones are normal, typically developing to approximately two years of age. Development then stagnates, and eventually all acquired motor activities deteriorate and are lost. Speech is lost entirely, sometimes within months of onset of the disorder.

Feeding Disorders: Initially, feeding is normal, but the onset of the disorder is marked by hypotonia followed by hyperactive reflexes, poor head control, abnormal posturing, and, finally, total loss of motor control, including gastrointestinal and esophageal function.

Voice Disorders: Initially, voice is normal, but at the onset of the degenerative process, hoarseness and breathiness are common.

Resonance Disorders: Initially resonance is normal. With the onset of neurological degeneration, hypernasality is likely to occur and become progressively more severe.

S

Language Disorders: Initially, language development is normal. Following the onset of the disorder, language stagnates and then degenerates until all useful language function is lost.

Other Clinical Features:

Central nervous system: CNS degeneration; brain swelling; axonal degeneration; seizures; hypotonia; abnormal reflexes;

Ocular: nystagmus; absence of tearing;

Endocrine: hypothyroidism; diabetes insipidus; lack of control of autonomic function, including temperature regulation;

Circulation: distal gangrene.

Natural History: Early development is normal, including all psychomotor milestones. The onset of observable symptoms is at approximately two years in many cases, but earlier symptoms have been observed. Within months of onset, significant neurological degeneration becomes evident with total loss of psychomotor milestones eventually occurring. Death occurs in nearly all cases within a decade of the onset of the initial findings.

Treatment Prognosis: The progression of the disorder cannot be halted and palliative treatment is not available.

Differential Diagnosis: The onset of a degenerative process in infancy or toddler years occurs in many of the lysosomal storage disorders, such as **Hurler syndrome** and **Hunter syndrome.** However, these disorders are characterized by significant progression of abnormal physical abnormalities related to intracellular storage of glycosaminoglycans.

SHORT Syndrome

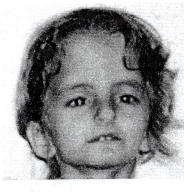

SHORT syndrome.

Also Known As: Short stature, lipoatrophy, and Rieger anomaly.

The appellation of SHORT syndrome is another attempt to match an acronym to one of the major findings associated with the disorder, as in **LEOPARD syndrome.** Short stature is one of the major findings in this multiple anomaly disorder, along with a distinctive facial appearance and Rieger anomaly, an ocular abnormality involving maldevelopment of the anterior chamber of the eye resulting in abnormal appearance of the iris and pupil.

Major System(s) Affected: Growth; craniofacial; ocular; musculoskeletal; dental; central nervous system.

Etiology: Autosomal recessive inheritance. The gene has not been mapped or identified.

Quick Clues: The association of subcutaneous wasting of fat with iris malformations (Rieger anomaly) is a distinctive association in SHORT syndrome.

Hearing Disorders: Sensorineural hearing loss is an occasional manifestation of the disorder.

Speech Disorders: Speech onset is delayed, usually more significantly than the degree of developmental delay would suggest. Articulation impairment is also common, related to delayed dental eruption and micrognathia.

Feeding Disorders: Feeding disorders have not been reported or observed.

Voice Disorders: Voice is typically high-pitched.

Resonance Disorders: Abnormal resonance characteristics have not been observed or reported.

Language Disorders: Language delay is common, with expressive language more impaired than receptive. The specific role of hearing impairment in relation to the language delay has not been determined, but because language impairment is a more common finding than hearing loss, it is likely that language impairment is a primary anomaly associated with the syndrome.

Other Clinical Features:

Growth: short stature; low birthweight; lipoatrophy;

Craniofacial: absence of facial fat; triangular facial shape; deep-set eyes; micrognathia;

downturned oral commissures;

Ocular: Rieger anomaly; anomalies of the iris and cornea; neonatal glaucoma;

Musculoskeletal: hyperextensible joints; congenital hip dislocation; inguinal hernia; delayed bone age;

Dental: delayed dental eruption;

Central nervous system: mild developmental delay.

Natural History: Mild developmental delay may be related to mild hypotonia and musculoskeletal weakness, but the severity of expressive language impairment makes the degree of psychomotor impairment look worse initially. With growth and age, the severity of lipoatrophy makes the children look increasingly dysmorphic, often giving them a prematurely aged appearance. Some cases have experienced chronic respiratory illness. Others have developed diabetes mellitus.

Treatment Prognosis: The prognosis is essentially good, and symptomatic and palliative treatments should be effective.

Differential Diagnosis: The facies is similar to that seen in Granddad syndrome, and has some similarities to **Bloom syndrome,** **Cockayne syndrome,** and progeria because of the prematurely aged appearance.

S

Spondyloepiphyseal Dysplasia Congenita

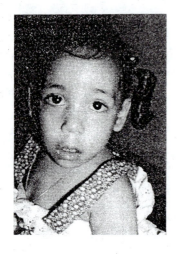

Spondyloepiphyseal dysplasia congenita.

Also Known As: SED; spondyloepiphyseal dysplasia.

Spondyloepiphyseal dysplasia congenita is a syndrome of short stature that can lead to Robin sequence, because micrognathia and cleft palate are common anomalies associated with the syndrome. The syndrome is caused by a mutation in the *COL2A1* gene, the same gene responsible for **Stickler syndrome**. The **Stickler** mutation, although in the same gene, is a different mutation in a different exon in the gene.

Major System(s) Affected: Growth; craniofacial; ocular; musculoskeletal; central nervous system.

Etiology: Autosomal dominant inheritance. The gene has been mapped to the long arm of chromosome 12 and has been identified as the *COL2A1* gene, a gene responsible for type 2 collagen formation.

Quick Clues: The flattened midface and mandibular deficiency associated with SED is distinctive when associated with short stature, although similar findings occur in **Kniest syndrome.**

Hearing Disorders: Sensorineural hearing loss is a common finding and is occasionally compounded by a conductive component secondary to chronic middle ear disease.

Speech Disorders: Articulation is often impaired, in part because of malocclusion, in part because of sensorineural hearing loss, and often related to compensatory substitutions secondary to cleft palate and velopharyngeal insufficiency.

Feeding Disorders: Infant feeding is often impaired by upper airway obstruction and cleft palate leading to failure-to-thrive.

Voice Disorders: Voice is typically high-pitched.

Resonance Disorders: Hypernasality secondary to cleft palate is common.

Language Disorders: Language development is often normal, but is impaired in the small percentage of cases with cognitive impairment.

Other Clinical Features:

> **Growth:** short stature, short trunk variety;

> **Craniofacial:** micrognathia; cleft palate; flat midface;

> **Ocular:** myopia; retinal detachment;

> **Musculoskeletal:** flattened vertebrae; short neck; cervical spine subluxation; odontoid hypoplasia; kyphoscoliosis; lumbar lordosis; pectus excavatum or carinatum;

> **Central nervous system:** occasional cognitive impairment.

Natural History: Skeletal anomalies are present at birth and growth deficiency becomes obvious early in life. Myopia is often congenital, but may not be detected until later in childhood. The myopia is progressive and vitreoretinal degeneration may result in retinal detachment. Hearing loss may also be progressive, especially in high frequencies.

Treatment Prognosis: The short stature is related to a primary skeletal dysplasia and, because it is of the short trunk variety, treatment is not possible at the present time. There is no contraindication to standard treatment for cleft palate. Feeding disorders can be resolved by treating the respiratory disorder, which rarely requires tracheotomy.

Differential Diagnosis: Diastrophic dysplasia syndrome is another syndrome of short stature, cleft palate, and Robin sequence. The skeletal abnormalities are different and can be detected by radiographs.

Steinert Syndrome

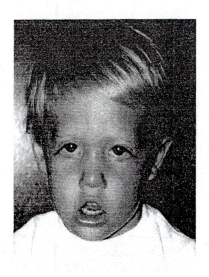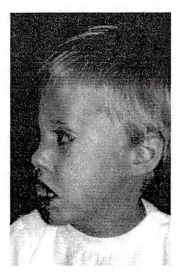

Steinert syndrome: Note myopathic facies, mouth-open posture, and vertical growth pattern.

Also Known As: Myotonic dystrophy.

Steinert syndrome is one of the more common forms of muscular dystrophy. The syndrome is interesting in genetic terms because it shows both anticipation and imprinting. Myotonic dystrophy affects all types of muscle (skeletal, smooth, and cardiac) so that speech and swallowing are both potentially impaired. When inherited from the mother, the disorder is expressed at birth and cognitive and language impairment are common.

Major System(s) Affected: Musculoskeletal; central nervous system; craniofacial; integument; ocular, genitourinary; gastrointestinal.

Etiology: Autosomal dominant inheritance. The disorder is one of a number of genetic disorders caused by an expansion of trinucleotide repeats, specifically a series of CTG repeats in a protein kinase gene mapped to 19q13.2-q13.3.

Quick Clues: Congenital cases are unmistakeable because of the severe myopathic facies that is present from birth. In cases with later onset, there are few physical manifestations early on, and perhaps the most indicative clue is speech deterioration of unknown origin.

Hearing Disorders: Sensorineural hearing loss is a common clinical manifestation of Steinert syndrome and may be moderate to severe and typically is progressive.

Speech Disorders: In congenital cases (maternally inherited), speech is severely delayed. Oral contacts are extremely weak and oral articulation extremely difficult. Few consonant sounds are recognizable. Lingual movements are severely impaired, and lip incompetence is the rule. In late-onset cases (paternally inherited), early speech development is normal and articulation is normal. Following onset (usually in the second decade of life), articulation may deteriorate, with mild dysarthria and weak oral contacts for pressure consonants.

Feeding Disorders: Feeding impairments with failure-to-thrive occurs only in the congenital form of Steinert syndrome. Swallowing is impaired because of involvement of smooth muscle as well as skeletal muscle. Weak oral movements prevent a lip seal around the nipple with poor or absent suction. Lower intestinal movements are also impaired, resulting in constipation and megacolon, thus creating an uncomfortable abdominal feeling and lack of appetite. In addition, muscle tone abnormalities result in upper airway obstruction and there is reduced pulmonary effort, thus further complicating feeding.

Voice Disorders: Breathy voice is common in the congenital form. In the late-onset form, voice is initially normal, but may eventually become breathy with progression of the myotonia.

Resonance Disorders: Hypernasality is common in both the congenital and late-onset forms of Steinert syndrome. In the congenital form, hypernasality is often present from the onset of speech. In the late-onset form, the spontaneous development of hypernasality is often the first presenting symptom of myotonic dystrophy. The hypernasality becomes progressively worse with advancement of the disorder.

Language Disorders: In the congenital form, language is delayed and impaired. The degree of impairment is variable, but in the most severe cases, language impairment can be very severe with expressive language more significantly affected than receptive.

Other Clinical Features:

Musculoskeletal: myotonia; progressive muscle wasting; club foot; thin ribs (congenital form);

Central nervous system: polyneuropathy; cognitive impairment (congenital form); personality change (late-onset form);

Craniofacial: vertical facial growth pattern with vertical maxillary excess secondary to lax facial musculature; eyelid ptosis; facial diplegia; Robin sequence (rare, in congenital form only);

Integument: male frontal balding in late onset form;

Ocular: cataracts; lens opacities;

Genitourinary: hypogonadism; urinary tract anomalies;

Gastrointestinal: megacolon; constipation;

Other: malignant hyperthermia in reponse to anesthesia.

Natural History: In the congenital form, the earliest signs of the syndrome occur during gestation. Mothers often note reduced fetal movement and may develop polyhydramnios. In the congenital form, muscle weakness is evident immediately and is severe, often with accompanying cognitive impairment and developmental delay. Speech is often the slowest of all developmental milestones. In the late-onset form, the spontaneous development of hypernasality is often one of the earliest findings, usually occurring in early adolescence. The disorder is always progressive.

Treatment Prognosis: All support therapies are indicated in the congenital form, but the more severe the expression, the less positive the response. In the late-onset form, support therapies are also indicated and have a better chance for a positive outcome. Because hypernasality is a common finding, there

S

may be referral for pharyngeal surgery, such as pharyngeal flap. However, many patients with Steinert syndrome respond to general anesthesia with a severe elevation of body temperature (malignant hyperthermia or hyperpyrexia) that can be potentially fatal. However, surgery can be performed success- fully if the anesthesiologist is prepared for the complication.

Differential Diagnosis: Muscle weakness and wasting are common manifestations of many muscular dystrophies. The differential diagnosis is dependent on muscle biopsy to determine the specific enzymatic abnormalities.

Stickler Syndrome

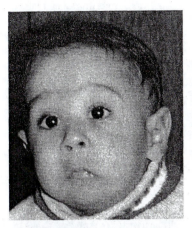
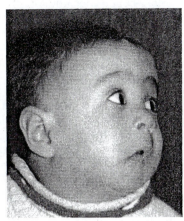

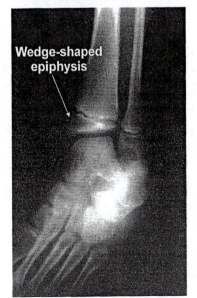

Wedge-shaped epiphysis

Stickler syndrome: Note the round facies, depressed nasal root, and micrognathia (top row). The epiphysis at the ankle is wedge-shaped (bottom).

S

Also Known As: Hereditary arthro-ophthalmopathy, Marshall-Stickler syndrome, Wagner-Stickler syndrome.

Stickler syndrome is one of the most common connective dysplasias in humans. Although much of the emphasis in Stickler syndrome has been on the ophthalmologic findings, hearing loss is a common finding and is often overlooked. Stickler syndrome is often encountered in craniofacial or cleft palate clinics because it is the most common syndrome that results in the Robin sequence. At least one-third of all babies initially diagnosed with Robin sequence have Stickler syndrome. The diagnosis can be difficult because most children with Stickler syndrome are normal in appearance, and the minor alterations they express in terms of craniofacial appearance are not particularly stigmatizing. Most children with Stickler syndrome could be called "cute" with round, cherubic faces. However, the syndrome has major impacts on speech, feeding, and hearing. The phenotype of what most clinicians label as Stickler syndrome is probably caused by more than one gene, all involved in the morphogenesis of collagen, a major component of cartilage and connective tissue. Because some skeletal structures are initially cartilaginous, eventual skeletal formation is also affected. The *COL2A1*, *COL11A1*, and *COL11A2* genes have all been implicated in producing the Stickler phenotype. It is unclear if the phenotypes caused by mutations in these separate genes are exactly the same, or simply close phenocopies.

Major System(s) Affected: Craniofacial; ocular; growth; musculoskeletal.

Etiology: Autosomal dominant inheritance. Several genes have been identified as possibly causing Stickler syndrome, including *COL2A1*, *COL11A1*, and *COL11A2*. *COL2A1* has been mapped to 12q13.11-q13.2. *COL11A1* has been mapped to 6p21.3 and *COL11A2* to 1p21. There are some variations in the phenotype depending on the specific gene causing the anomalies. Hearing loss, more specifically sensorineural impairment, is specific to the *COL2A1* and *COL11A1* mutations. The candidate genes for Stickler syndrome are responsible for formation of collagen, a major component of connective tissue and cartilage. Different mutations in this same gene cause **spondyloepiphyseal dysplasia congenita** and **Kniest syndrome.**

Quick Clues: A child who is wearing very thick glasses for myopia and has a high frequency sensorineural hearing loss, or who may have cleft palate and thick lenses is highly likely to have Stickler syndrome.

Hearing Disorders: Sensorineural hearing loss, usually in the high frequencies, is found in at least 15% of patients with Stickler syndrome, but some reports have cited a frequency of nearly 80%. The sensorineural hearing loss may be progressive, especially in the high frequencies. Conductive loss secondary to chronic middle ear effusion is also common, especially among those cases with cleft palate.

Speech Disorders: Articulation disorders secondary to malocclusion are common. Micrognathia, with or without anterior skeletal open-bite, is a common finding in Stickler syndrome resulting in lingual-protrusion distortions. In cases with severe micrognathia, tongue-backing may occur. Compensatory articulation patterns secondary to cleft palate and velopharyngeal insufficiency should be expected in some cases.

Feeding Disorders: Early neonatal respiratory distress and upper airway obstruction often leads to feeding disorders. Failure-to-thrive in Stickler syndrome is solely related to upper airway obstruction, often the product of glossoptosis. A short genioglossus muscle and lingual attachment in the mandible restricts anterior tongue movement.

Voice Disorders: Voice production is typically normal in Stickler syndrome.

Resonance Disorders: Hypernasality secondary to cleft palate is an occasional finding. Hyponasality, or cul-de-sac resonance, has also been observed in cases with an extremely small nasal cavity or small nostrils.

Language Disorders: Language development is typically normal in Stickler syndrome, as is cognitive development.

Other Clinical Features:

> **Craniofacial:** micrognathia; cleft palate; Robin sequence; acute angulation of the cranial base; short ramus with normal condyles; antegonial notching of the body of the mandible; maxillary hypo-

plasia; depressed nasal root; round face; epicanthal folds;

Ocular: myopia, often congenital and severe; vitreoretinal degeneration; retinal detachment resulting in blindness; occasional cataracts;

Growth: occasional short stature; occasional tall stature;

Musculoskeletal: lax joints; epiphyseal dysplasia; osteochondrodysplasia; spondyloepiphyseal dysplasia; joint pains, especially in the knees or lower back.

Natural History: Hearing loss may be detected late because the most common presentation is a mild to moderate sensorineural loss in the high frequencies. No data are available to determine if newborn otoacoustic emission screening or newborn brainstem testing has been successful in identifying such cases. Many babies with Stickler syndrome are born with Robin sequence, constituting approximately one-third of all babies with Robin. Micrognathia may be severe at birth resulting in respiratory and feeding disorders with failure-to-thrive. With age, the maxilla and mandible often become proportionate leading some clinicians to believe that the mandible is exhibiting "catch-up growth." However, the situation is such that the mandible is not really growing so much as the maxilla is hypoplastic. Some children with Stickler syndrome are initially thought to be hypotonic, but in most cases, joint hyperextensibility is related to connective tissue dysplasia rather than true hypotonia. The early presentation of myopia is common, but not universal, in the syndrome and the visual impairment is typically progressive.

Treatment Prognosis: Excellent. Amplification is indicated in those cases with significant hearing loss. In cases with cleft palate, vigorous otologic follow-up is essential. With proper care, severe eye problems can be avoided. Cleft palate repair is typically successful. Orthognathic surgery is not typically necessary, but is not contraindicated when micrognathia persists.

Differential Diagnosis: Robin sequence and eye problems also occur in **SED congenita (spondyloepiphyseal dysplasia),** but short stature in **SED** is far more pronounced. **Kniest syndrome,** also caused by a mutation in *COL2A1* has a similar facial phenotype, but more severe short stature and marked distortion of the thorax. Isolated (nonsyndromic) Robin sequence has a very similar presentation at birth, but does not have joint or ocular problems as associated findings.

Townes-Brocks Syndrome

Also Known As: Townes syndrome.

The association of facial, ear, rectal, renal, and limb anomalies with hearing loss was delineated as an entity separate from **oculo-auriculo-vertebral spectrum (OAVS)** in the 1970s. It is likely that some individuals with Townes-Brocks syndrome have been mistakenly diagnosed as having **OAVS**.

Major System(s) Affected: Craniofacial; musculoskeletal; gastrointestinal; genitourinary; cardiac; central nervous system.

Etiology: Autosomal dominant inheritance. The gene has been mapped to 16q12.1 and the gene is thought to be *SALL1* putative transcription factor.

Quick Clues: The presence of triphalangeal thumbs with anomalous external ears and a history of imperforate anus should raise the suspicion of the diagnosis of Townes-Brocks syndrome.

Hearing Disorders: Sensorineural hearing loss predominates, but conductive elements may also be present, resulting in a mixed loss. Ossicular anomalies are found in some cases. Severity is variable, but does not seem to be progressive. Ear anomalies and hearing loss may be unilateral or bilateral.

Speech Disorders: Speech may be affected by the hearing loss if it is bilaterally severe or profound.

Feeding Disorders: Early feeding in infancy may be affected by anal stenosis or imperforate anus, resulting in slow clearing of the bowel.

Voice Disorders: Voice is normal.

Resonance Disorders: Resonance is typically normal, although the author has seen one patient with Townes-Brocks syndrome with cleft palate.

Language Disorders: Language development is typically normal.

Other Clinical Features:

> **Craniofacial:** external ear anomalies; ear tags or pits; microtia;

Musculoskeletal: triphalangeal thumbs; hypoplastic and low-set thumbs; supernumerary thumbs; syndactyly; clinodactyly; absent bones in the hands or feet; radial anomalies;

Gastrointestinal: anal stenosis or imperforate anus; rectoperineal fistula;

Genitourinary: rectovaginal fistula; hypoplastic/aplastic kidney;

Cardiac: ventriculoseptal defect,

Central nervous system: occasional cognitive impairment.

Natural History: The anomalies associated with the syndrome, including the hearing loss, are static and essentially nonprogressive.

Treatment Prognosis: The prognosis is good with all the anomalies other than the occasionally observed cognitive impairment which is surgically correctable.

Differential Diagnosis: The association of hearing loss with asymmetric or malformed ears and ear tags or pits is commonly found in **oculo-auriculo-vertebral spectrum disorder.** Ear pits and hearing loss with kidney anomalies is seen in **BOR syndrome.**

Treacher Collins Syndrome

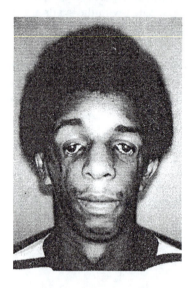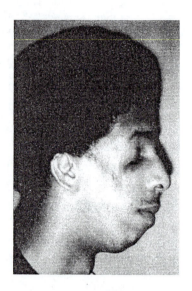

Treacher Collins syndrome: Note the downslanting eyes, malar depressions, micrognathia, and the projection of hair onto the cheek.

Also Known As: mandibulofacial dysostosis; Franceschetti-Klein syndrome, Franceschetti-Zwahlen-Klein syndrome.

Treacher Collins syndrome, named for 19th century ophthalmologist Edward Treacher Collins, has been recognized as a distinct multiple anomaly disorder for over 150 years. Though relatively rare, the syndrome has such a distinctive ap-

pearance that it is one of the most easily recognized of craniofacial syndromes. There are no extracranial anomalies associated with Treacher Collins syndrome, although some have been reported. It is likely that some patients have other common anomalies, including congenital heart malformations (such as VSD) in association with the syndrome as a chance and coincidental occurrence. Treacher

Collins syndrome is widely regarded as having a population prevalence of 1:10,000. Expression is highly variable, and some affected individuals are quite normal in appearance, while others have severe craniofacial malformations.

Major System(s) Affected:
Craniofacial.

Etiology: Autosomal dominant inheritance. The gene has been mapped to 5q32-q33.1 and has been labeled the *TREACLE* gene.

Quick Clues: Microtia is most often a unilateral malformation, but in the very large majority of cases of Treacher Collins syndrome, microtia is bilateral and symmetric. Also of note is the absence of eyelashes on the inner third of the lower eyelid. This eyelash anomaly in association with conductive hearing loss should raise the suspicion of Treacher Collins syndrome.

Hearing Disorders: Probably the most common clinical feature of the syndrome is conductive hearing loss. Even patients with very mild facial manifestations of Treacher Collins syndrome have conductive hearing loss. Fixation of the footplate of the stapes is common even when the ossicles and middle ear are intact. Maximal conductive hearing loss is common because Grade II and Grade III microtia are common anomalies. Complete atresia of the middle ear and ossicles is common.

Speech Disorders: Articulation is commonly impaired in Treacher Collins syndrome in a number of ways. In some cases, the severe micrognathia causes persistent tongue-backing with multiple substitutions for anterior sounds (such as bilabials, lingua-alveolars, and lingua-dentals) with posterior sounds, including compensatory maneuvers, such as pharyngeal stops, laryngeal stops, and pharyngeal fricatives. Also common are anterior distortions secondary to anterior skeletal open-bite, a frequent anomaly in the syndrome. Cleft palate, sometimes near absence of the palate, can contribute to additional abnormal compensations, including glottal stops.

Feeding Disorders: Early feeding problems and failure-to-thrive are very common manifestations of Treacher Collins syndrome in the neonatal period and infancy and are related to airway obstruction. Airway obstruction has a number of etiologies, including choanal atresia or stenosis, micrognathia,

Robin sequence, and pharyngeal hypoplasia. Babies with Treacher Collins often have severe upper airway obstruction as soon as they close their mouths. Resolution of the airway problems allows normal feeding.

Voice Disorders: Voice is typically normal in Treacher Collins syndrome.

Resonance Disorders: Resonance disorders are very common and of unusual type in Treacher Collins syndrome. Hypernasality is possible in cases with cleft palate or cleft lip and palate. However, because the entire pharynx is very small in diameter, hypernasality is much less common than hyponasality or mixed resonance. In cases of mixed resonance, it is common to find hyponasality with occasional nasal turbulence and nasal emission. Oral resonance is often severely impaired by retrodisplacement of the tongue and a hypoplastic pharyngeal airway. Oral resonance is muffled with marked damping of sound that would normally resonate in the oropharynx and nasopharynx. Even normal sized tonsils can further impair oral resonance characteristics. Oral resonance and nasal resonance abnormalities are not mutually exclusive and may coexist.

Language Disorders: Language is almost always normal in Treacher Collins syndrome, as is intellect, unless there has been severe neonatal hypoxia with subsequent hypoxic brain damage.

Other Clinical Features:

> **Craniofacial:** downslanting palpebral fissures; clefting or absence of the zygomas; malar bone clefting; bony orbital clefts; micrognathia, often very severe; antegonial notching of the mandible; acute cranial base angle; notch in the lower eyelid; absence of eyelashes on the inner third of the eye; absent puncta; lacrimal duct stenosis or obstruction; microtia; cleft palate; cleft lip and palate (less common than cleft palate alone); projection of hair onto the cheek; absence of angle between the nasal bridge and the forehead; anterior skeletal open-bite.

Natural History: The anomalies associated with Treacher Collins syndrome are all present at birth and there is no progression. Upper airway obstruction may not be obvious initially, but is often present within the first few days of life. In cases with more severe craniofacial manifestations, airway obstruction is immediate after birth.

Treatment Prognosis: All structural anomalies in Treacher Collins syndrome can be treated surgically, and in many cases, outcomes can be very good. Osseous distraction is a new tool being used for severe micrognathia early in life. The palatal clefts can often be difficult to repair because of a severe tissue deficiency, but hypernasality may not be a problem, even in cases with severe palatal anomalies. The airway obstruction is so severe in some cases that tracheotomy becomes necessary. Bone conduction hearing aids are indicated in cases with severe microtia, but in less severe microtia, it may be possible to use air conduction aids. Caution needs to be exercised in reconstructive surgery in the middle ear because of an anomalous course of the VIIth cranial nerve, which may course through the footplate of the stapes.

Differential Diagnosis: In the earlier years of the delineation of Treacher Collins syndrome, the disorder was often grouped together with **oculo-auriculo-vertebral dysplasia,** thought to be a unilateral expression of the same disorder. **Miller syndrome** has similar craniofacial manifestations, but has unusual limb anomalies. Probably most similar to Treacher Collins syndrome is **Nager syndrome,** which has very similar craniofacial anomalies, but also has thumb and radial anomalies not found in Treacher Collins syndrome.

Turner Syndrome

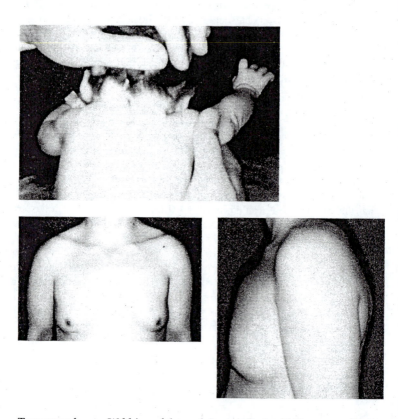

Turner syndrome: Webbing of the neck in an infant with Turner syndrome (top). Abnormal breast development and "shield-shaped chest" in an adult with mosaic Turner syndrome (bottom).

Also Known As: XO syndrome; 45, X syndrome; monosomy X; Morgagni-Turner-Albright syndrome; Schereshevkii-Turner syndrome; Bonnevie-Ulrich syndrome; Turner-Varny syndrome.

Turner syndrome is a relatively common multiple anomaly syndrome, with a population prevalence of approximately 1:2,500. All affected individuals are phenotypically female because the disorder is caused by absence of one of the sex chromosomes, leaving a single X chromosome (sex chromosome or X chromosome monosomy). Many cases are mosaics, meaning that not all the cells in the body have 45X karytoypes. The larger the percentage of cells missing the X chromosome, the more severe the expression of the disorder. In cases that have 100% of cells with an X chromosome monosomy, there is absence of secondary sexual characteristics, absence of gonads, and short stature. Webbing of the neck is variable.

Major System(s) Affected:
Growth; genitourinary; craniofacial; musculoskeletal; limbs; integument; cardiac; central nervous system; endocrine; ocular.

Etiology: Deletion of one copy of the X chromosome from all or some of the cells in the body.

Quick Clues: Webbing of the neck and short stature in females is a strong indication of Turner syndrome. However, mosaic cases show less severe expressions of these features, and in some cases, webbing of the neck is absent or difficult to notice.

Hearing Disorders: Sensorineural hearing loss is found in approximately half of individuals with Turner syndrome. In some cases, chronic middle ear disease may result in a mixed loss.

Speech Disorders: Articulation impairment secondary to malocclusion is common, including lingual protrusion secondary to anterior skeletal open-bite, and in some cases, tongue-backing secondary to micrognathia. Speech onset is often delayed.

Feeding Disorders: Early failure-to-thrive may occur secondary to airway obstruction, micrognathia, and/or Robin sequence.

Voice Disorders: Hoarseness is common, as is a high-pitched voice in some cases.

Resonance Disorders: Hypernasality secondary to cleft palate or submucous cleft palate is common.

Language Disorders: Language impairment, especially in terms of expressive language, is common, although cognitive impairment is not a common finding in the syndrome. Nearly all patients have normal intellect, but learning disorders are relatively common, usually in the areas of mathematics and spatial relationships. These problems are usually relatively minor.

Other Clinical Features:

Growth: short stature;

Genitourinary: gonadal aplasia (in complete monosomies) or hypoplasia (in mosaicism); kidney anomalies;

Craniofacial: cleft palate (often submucous); micrognathia; malocclusion; epicanthi; low-set posteriorly rotated ears; prominent ears; low posterior hairline;

Musculoskeletal: broad (shield-shaped) chest resulting in wide-spaced nipples; hip dislocation; scoliosis; skeletal dysplaisa;

Limbs: cubitus valgus; spoon-shaped nails; short fourth metatarsal and metacarpal; knee anomalies;

Integument: multiple pigmented nevi; tendency to form keloid scars; webbing of the neck (pterygium colli);

Cardiac: aortic valve anomalies, coarctation of the aorta;

Central nervous system: learning disabilities;

Endocrine: absence or incomplete development of secondary sexual characteristics; diabetes mellitus; thyroid disorders;

Ocular: cataracts; strabismus; ptosis.

Natural History: The major anomalies associated with Turner syndrome are typically evident at birth in cases of complete monosomies. In patients with mosaicisms, anomalies may be minor, almost unnoticeable in many cases. The first indications of the diagnosis in such cases may be primary amenorrhea and delayed or absent development of secondary sexual characteristics. Life expectancy is not known to be impaired.

Treatment Prognosis: Symptomatic treatments are effective, including the use of growth hormone and estrogen replacement. Speech therapy, palatal surgery, and orthognathic surgery are all indicated, as is language therapy in those cases with impairment.

Differential Diagnosis: Noonan syndrome when present in females has many similar features, although the heart anomalies are different. Some patients with **velo-cardio-facial syndrome** have webbing of the neck together with retrognathia, cleft palate, and mild growth deficiency. Karyotype will differentiate the syndromes.

Usher Syndrome, Type IA

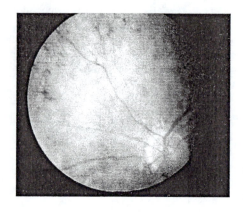

Usher syndrome: Retinitis pigmentosa on examination of the retina in Usher syndrome, type IA.

Also Known As: Retinitis pigmentosa and sensorineural hearing loss.

Although the association of retinitis pigmentosa (RP) and sensorineural hearing loss is referred to in aggregate as Usher syndrome, there are actually a number of separate and distinct syndromes that have been labeled as subtypes. These subtypes have varying phenotypes and multiple etiologies, so the inclusion of all of these disorders under the term "Usher syndrome" is nosologically somewhat confusing; the grouping together of these multiple genetic entities under one eponym acknowledges the early contributions of Charles Usher in 1914.

Three broad types of Usher syndrome have been described according to the onset of the visual and hearing symptoms. Type I is characterized by profound sensorineural hearing loss at birth and the subsequent development of RP before 10 years of age. Type II is a milder expression with a less severe form of congenital sensorineural hearing loss and a later onset of RP, usually in late teen years. Type III shows progressive sensorineural hearing loss with the onset of RP in the early teens (usually at or near puberty). A fourth type, presumed to be X-linked, has been hypothesized, but is most likely autosomal recessive and not a distinct diagnostic entity. In type IA, a variety of cells derived from ciliated precursor cells are impaired. These include the hair cells in the cochlea and vestibular aparatus, photoreceptor cells, and nasal hair cells. Low sperm motility has also been noted leading to decreased fertility in affected males. When all subtypes of Usher syndrome are totaled, these disorders account for over half of all people who are deaf and blind.

Major System(s) Affected:
Auditory; vestibular; ocular; central nervous system.

Etiology: Autosomal recessive inheritance. The gene has been mapped to 14q32.

Quick Clues: There are no external physical manifestations in any of the Usher syndromes. The association of sensorineural hearing loss and visual impairment should point towards this disorder, and type IA is particularly suspect when clumsy gait is present.

Hearing Disorders: Profound bilateral sensorineural hearing loss is present at birth. Vestibular function is impaired, often resulting in clumsy gait and occasional ataxia.

Speech Disorders: "Deaf speech" occurs in nearly all cases.

Feeding Disorders: Feeding disorders are not associated with the Usher syndromes.

Voice Disorders: Vocal production is impaired only as a result of hearing loss.

Resonance Disorders: Muffled oral resonance with mixed hyper-/hyponasality (consistent with "deaf speech."

Language Disorders: Verbal language development is impaired by congenital hearing loss.

Other Clinical Features:

Ocular: retinitis pigmentosa; cataracts;

Central nervous system: cognitive impairment; psychiatric illness; ataxia.

Natural History: Hearing loss is congenital with RP developing in late childhood, usually by 10 years of age. Central nervous system impairments are congenital.

Treatment Prognosis: Palliative treatment is the only possible treatment at this time and the prognosis for improvement in hearing or vision is limited.

Differential Diagnosis: The various subtypes of the Usher syndromes all show some degree of visual impairment and hearing loss. **Refsum syndrome** also has this association along with degenerative polyneuritis and metabolic abnormalities.

Usher Syndrome, Type IB

Also Known As: Usher syndrome, non-Acadian variety; myosin VIIA.

Usher syndrome, type IB is similar in phenotype to IA.

Major System(s) Affected: Auditory; vestibular; ocular; central nervous system.

Etiology: Autosomal recessive inheritance. The gene has been mapped to 11q13.5. A number of different mutations in the same gene have been described. The various mutations in this gene cause abnormalities in the gene encoding myosin VIIA. Degeneration of the hair cells of the cochlea results from the abnormal protein product of this gene.

Quick Clues: There are no external physical manifestations in any of the Usher syndromes. The association of sensorineural hearing loss and progressive visual impairment with psychiatric disturbance and ataxia should point towards one of the type I forms of Usher syndrome.

Hearing Disorders: Profound bilateral sensorineural hearing loss is present at birth. Vestibular function is impaired.

Speech Disorders: "Deaf speech" occurs in nearly all cases.

Feeding Disorders: Feeding disorders are not associated with the Usher syndromes.

Voice Disorders: Vocal production is impaired only as a result of hearing loss.

Resonance Disorders: Muffled oral resonance with mixed hyper-/hyponasality (consistent with "deaf speech."

Language Disorders: Verbal language development is impaired by congenital hearing loss.

Other Clinical Features:

> **Ocular:** progressive retinitis pigmentosa; blindness; cataracts;

Central nervous system: cognitive impairment; psychosis; ataxia.

Natural History: Hearing loss is congenital with RP developing in childhood before 10 years of age. Central nervous system impairments are congenital.

Treatment Prognosis: Palliative treatment is the only possible treatment at this time and the prognosis for improvement in hearing or vision is limited.

Differential Diagnosis: The various subtypes of the Usher syndromes all show some degree of visual impairment and hearing loss. **Refsum syndrome** also has this association along with degenerative polyneuritis and metabolic abnormalities.

Usher Syndrome, Type IC

Also Known As: Usher syndrome, Acadian variety.

Usher syndrome, type IC is similar in phenotype to IA, but is most commonly found in the Acadian (Cajun) population of southwestern Louisiana and their descendants.

Major System(s) Affected: Auditory; vestibular; ocular; central nervous system.

Etiology: Autosomal recessive inheritance. The gene has been mapped to 11p15.1.

Quick Clues: There are no external physical manifestations in any of the Usher syndromes. The association of sensorineural hearing loss and progressive visual in someone of Acadian (Cajun) descent should make the diagnosis highly likely.

Hearing Disorders: Profound bilateral sensorineural hearing loss is present at birth. Vestibular function is impaired.

Speech Disorders: "Deaf speech" occurs in nearly all cases.

Feeding Disorders: Feeding disorders are not associated with the Usher syndromes.

Voice Disorders: Vocal production is impaired only as a result of hearing loss.

Resonance Disorders: Muffled oral resonance with mixed hyper-/hyponasality (consistent with "deaf speech."

Language Disorders: Verbal language development is impaired by congenital hearing loss.

Other Clinical Features:

> **Ocular:** progressive retinitis pigmentosa; blindness; cataracts;

> **Central nervous system:** cognitive impairment; psychosis; ataxia.

Natural History: Hearing loss is congenital with RP developing in childhood before 10 years of age. Central nervous system impairments are congenital.

U

Treatment Prognosis: Palliative treatment is the only possible treatment at this time and the prognosis for improvement in hearing or vision is limited.

Differential Diagnosis: The various subtypes of the Usher syndromes all show some degree of visual impairment and hearing loss. **Refsum syndrome** also has this association along with degenerative polyneuritis and metabolic abnormalities.

Usher Syndrome, Type ID

Also Known As:

Usher syndrome, type ID is similar in phenotype to IA, IB, and IC, but was found in Pakistanis.

Major System(s) Affected: Auditory; vestibular; ocular; central nervous system.

Etiology: Autosomal recessive inheritance. The gene has been mapped to 10q.

Quick Clues: There are no external physical manifestations in any of the Usher syndromes. The association of sensorineural hearing loss and progressive visual impairment in Pakistani individuals should lead to the suspicion of Usher syndrome, type ID.

Hearing Disorders: Profound bilateral sensorineural hearing loss is present at birth. Vestibular function is impaired.

Speech Disorders: "Deaf speech" occurs in nearly all cases.

Feeding Disorders: Feeding disorders are not associated with the Usher syndromes.

Voice Disorders: Vocal production is impaired only as a result of hearing loss.

Resonance Disorders: Muffled oral resonance with mixed hyper-/hyponasality (consistent with "deaf speech."

Language Disorders: Verbal language development is impaired by congenital hearing loss.

Other Clinical Features:

> **Ocular:** progressive retinitis pigmentosa; blindness; cataracts;

> **Central nervous system:** cognitive impairment; psychosis; ataxia.

Natural History: Hearing loss is congenital with RP developing in childhood before 10 years of age. Central nervous system impairments are congenital.

Treatment Prognosis: Palliative treatment is the only possible treatment at this time and the prognosis for improvement in hearing or vision is limited.

U

Differential Diagnosis: The various subtypes of the Usher syndromes all show some degree of visual impairment and hearing loss. **Refsum syndrome** also has this association along with degenerative polyneuritis and metabolic abnormalities.

Usher Syndrome, Type IE

Also Known As:

Usher syndrome, type IE is similar in phenotype to IA, IB, and IC, but was found in Moroccan kindreds.

Major System(s) Affected:
Auditory; vestibular; ocular.

Etiology: Autosomal recessive
inheritance. The gene has been mapped to 21q21.

Quick Clues: There are no external physical manifestations in any of the Usher syndromes. The association of sensorineural hearing loss and progressive visual impairment in Moroccan individuals should lead to the suspicion of Usher syndrome, type IE.

Hearing Disorders: Profound
bilateral sensorineural hearing loss is present at birth. Vestibular function is impaired.

Speech Disorders: "Deaf
speech" occurs in nearly all cases.

Feeding Disorders: Feeding
disorders are not associated with the Usher syndromes.

Voice Disorders: Vocal production is impaired only as a result of hearing loss.

Resonance Disorders: Muffled oral resonance with mixed hyper-/hyponasality (consistent with "deaf speech."

Language Disorders: Verbal
language development is impaired by congenital hearing loss.

Other Clinical Features:

> **Ocular:** progressive retinitis pigmentosa; blindness; cataracts;

> **Vestibular:** ataxia.

Natural History: Hearing loss is
congenital with RP developing in childhood before 10 years of age. Central nervous system impairments are congenital.

Treatment Prognosis: Palliative treatment is the only possible treatment at this time and the prognosis for improvement in hearing or vision is limited.

U

Differential Diagnosis: The various subtypes of the Usher syndromes all show some degree of visual impairment and hearing loss. **Refsum syndrome** also has this association along with degenerative polyneuritis and metabolic abnormalities.

Usher Syndrome, Type IF

Also Known As:

Usher syndrome, type IF is similar in phenotype to IA, IB, and IC, but was found in Hutterite kindreds.

Major System(s) Affected: Auditory; vestibular; ocular.

Etiology: Autosomal recessive inheritance. The gene has been mapped to chromosome 10.

Quick Clues: There are no external physical manifestations in any of the Usher syndromes. The association of sensorineural hearing loss and progressive visual impairment in Hutterite individuals should lead to the suspicion of Usher syndrome, type IF.

Hearing Disorders: Profound bilateral sensorineural hearing loss is present at birth. Vestibular function is impaired.

Speech Disorders: "Deaf speech" occurs in nearly all cases.

Feeding Disorders: Feeding disorders are not associated with the Usher syndromes.

Voice Disorders: Vocal production is impaired only as a result of hearing loss.

Resonance Disorders: Muffled oral resonance with mixed hyper-/hyponasality (consistent with "deaf speech."

Language Disorders: Verbal language development is impaired by congenital hearing loss.

Other Clinical Features:

>**Ocular:** progressive retinitis pigmentosa; blindness; cataracts;

>**Vestibular:** ataxia.

Natural History: Hearing loss is congenital with RP developing in childhood before 10 years of age. Central nervous system impairments are congenital.

Treatment Prognosis: Palliative treatment is the only possible treatment at this time and the prognosis for improvement in hearing or vision is limited.

U

Differential Diagnosis: The various subtypes of the Usher syndromes all show some degree of visual impairment and hearing loss. **Refsum syndrome** also has this association along with degenerative polyneuritis and metabolic abnormalities.

Usher Syndrome, Type IIA

Also Known As:

Usher syndrome, type IIA differs from the type I Usher syndromes in that the onset of the retinitis pigmentosa is later and the progression slower. The hearing loss is also less severe and is not necessarily congenital with an onset in childhood.

Major System(s) Affected: Auditory; ocular.

Etiology: Autosomal recessive inheritance. The gene has been mapped to 1q41. Several different mutations in the same gene have been identified.

Quick Clues: There are no external physical manifestations in any of the Usher syndromes. The association of moderate to severe sensorineural hearing loss and progressive visual impairment beginning in teen years should lead to the suspicion of Usher syndrome, type II.

Hearing Disorders: Moderate to severe bilateral sensorineural hearing loss is detected during childhood. Vestibular function is not impaired.

Speech Disorders: Speech may be affected by sensorineural hearing loss if the impairment is not detected early and managed properly.

Feeding Disorders: Feeding disorders are not associated with the Usher syndromes.

Voice Disorders: Vocal production is normal.

Resonance Disorders: Resonance is normal unless the hearing loss remains undetected.

Language Disorders: Verbal language development may be impaired by hearing loss.

Other Clinical Features:

>**Ocular:** progressive retinitis pigmentosa.

Natural History: RP develops in teen years.

Treatment Prognosis: Amplification is indicated. The RP is of

U

later onset and slower progression, but definitive treatment is not available.

Differential Diagnosis: The various subtypes of the Usher syndromes all show some degree of visual impairment and hearing loss. **Refsum syndrome** also has this association along with degenerative polyneuritis and metabolic abnormalities.

Usher Syndrome, Type IIB

Also Known As:

Usher syndrome, type IIB differs from the type I Usher syndromes in that the onset of the retinitis pigmentosa is later and the progression slower. The hearing loss is also less severe.

Major System(s) Affected:
Auditory; ocular.

Etiology: Autosomal recessive inheritance. The gene has been mapped to 3p24.3-p23.

Quick Clues: There are no external physical manifestations in any of the Usher syndromes. The association of moderate to severe sensorineural hearing loss and progressive visual impairment beginning in teen years should lead to the suspicion of Usher syndrome, type IIB.

Hearing Disorders: Moderate to severe bilateral sensorineural hearing loss is detected during childhood. Vestibular function is not impaired.

Speech Disorders: Speech may be affected by sensorineural hearing loss if the impairment is not detected early and managed properly.

Feeding Disorders: Feeding disorders are not associated with the Usher syndromes.

Voice Disorders: Vocal production is normal.

Resonance Disorders: Resonance is normal unless the hearing loss remains undetected.

Language Disorders: Verbal language development may be impaired by hearing loss.

Other Clinical Features:

> **Ocular:** progressive retinitis pigmentosa.

Natural History: RP develops in teen years.

Treatment Prognosis: Amplification is indicated. The RP is of later onset and slower progression, but definitive treatment is not available.

Differential Diagnosis: The various subtypes of the Usher syndromes all show some degree of visual impairment and hearing loss. **Refsum syndrome** also has this association along with degenerative polyneuritis and metabolic abnormalities.

Usher Syndrome, Type III

Also Known As:

Usher syndrome, type III differs from the type II Usher syndromes in that there are vestibular manifestations and central nervous system abnormalities. The hearing loss is progressive. This form of Usher syndrome is most common among the Finnish population, but it is also found in the Acadian population of Western Louisiana, as are both type I and type II Usher syndrome.

Major System(s) Affected:
Auditory; ocular; central nervous system.

Etiology:
Autosomal recessive inheritance. The gene has been mapped to 3p24.3-p23.

Quick Clues:
There are no external physical manifestations in any of the Usher syndromes. The association of moderate to progressive sensorineural hearing loss and progressive visual impairment with neurologic symptoms should lead to the suspicion of Usher syndrome, type III.

Hearing Disorders:
Progressive bilateral sensorineural hearing loss. Vestibular function is also impaired.

Speech Disorders:
Speech is not as severely affected early in life because hearing is initially relatively normal and sensorineural hearing loss becomes more severe later in life. However, speech may deteriorate later with the onset of neurologic symptoms.

Feeding Disorders:
Feeding disorders are not associated with the Usher syndromes.

Voice Disorders:
Vocal production is normal.

Resonance Disorders:
Resonance is initially normal but may deteriorate with the onset of neurologic symptoms.

Language Disorders:
Verbal language development may be impaired by hearing loss. There may be deterioration later in life as neurologic symptoms progress.

Other Clinical Features:

Ocular: progressive retinitis pigmentosa;

U

Central Nervous System: cognitive impairment, ataxia; psychiatric illness.

Natural History: RP and neurologic symptoms develop in late teen years and are progressive.

Treatment Prognosis: Amplification is indicated. The onset of RP and neurologic symptoms have no effective treatment at this time.

Differential Diagnosis: The various subtypes of the Usher syndromes all show some degree of visual impairment and hearing loss. **Refsum syndrome** also has this association along with degenerative polyneuritis and metabolic abnormalities.

Van Buchem Syndrome

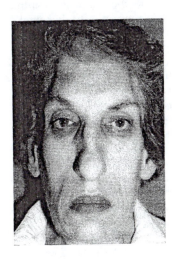

Van Buchem syndrome: Bony overgrowth of the face in van Buchem syndrome.

Also Known As: Van Buchem disease; generalized cortical hyperostosis; hyperphosphatasemia tarda; endosteal hyperostosis; sclerosteosis (thought by some to be the same disorder, while other clinicians believe this to be a separate, but similar syndrome).

Van Buchem syndrome is an autosomal recessive disorder of bony overgrowth that generally shows a late onset of clinical findings, although it is probable that the actual process begins early in life. The disorder has most often been reported in people of Dutch descent, including South Africans of Dutch ancestry. It has been suggested that van Buchem syndrome and a disorder known as sclerosteosis represent the same disorder. Sclerosteosis has also been reported primarily in individuals of Dutch descent, including South Africans (Afrikaners). The skeletal findings in van Buchem syndrome and sclerosteosis are essentially the same, but sclerosteosis has been described as being more severe and involving syndactyly of the second and third fingers. However, these findings may represent

291

variable expression of the same disorder. Therefore, there will not be a separate entry for sclerosteosis.

Major System(s) Affected:
Craniofacial; skeletal; central nervous system; ocular.

Etiology:
Autosomal recessive inheritance. The gene has been mapped to 17q11.2.

Quick Clues:
The first visible change is often progressive increase in size of the mandible, typically at an age later than the normal mandibular growth spurt.

Hearing Disorders:
Progressive hearing loss is a nearly constant finding. The hearing loss is typically mixed at first, progressing to a profound sensorineural hearing loss related to compression of the auditory nerve. Hyperostoses of the ossicles and progressive otosclerosis can also contribute to a moderate to severe conductive component. Fixed and fused ossicles are common. The onset of hearing loss is typically in the teen years.

Speech Disorders:
Initially, speech is normal. As bony overgrowth becomes more severe, the cranial nerves become compressed. Dysarthria becomes progressive. Prior to the onset of dysarthria, articulation may be impaired by progressive bony overgrowth that results in abnormalities of jaw structure, which may result in malocclusion and obligatory placement errors. Facial paresthesia may exacerbate the problem.

Feeding Disorders:
Early feeding is not impaired. Later in life, continuous compression of the cranial nerves, the spinal cord, and brainstem can lead to dysphagia. There is some loss of sensation in the facial musculature.

Voice Disorders:
Voice is initially normal, and then becomes progressively hoarse or breathy with restricted motion of the vocal cords, probably related to progressive sclerosis of the laryngeal cartilages.

Resonance Disorders:
Hyponasality secondary to nasal obstruction may develop late in life.

Language Disorders:
Language development is normal.

Other Clinical Features:

Craniofacial: progressive enlargement of the mandible with occasional asymmetry, often appearing square at the chin; exorbitism; mild hypertelorism; skeletal overgrowth resulting in closure of the cranial foramina, including the optic foramen and compression of the auditory nerve; thickening of the calvarium; progressive facial paresis;

Skeletal: diaphyseal thickening of the long bones; cortical hyperostosis;

Central nervous system: headaches; progressive increase of intracranial pressure; compression of the cranial nerves; anosmia;

Ocular: progressive optic atrophy; strabismus; occasional blindness.

Natural History: There is significant variability of expression, but in many of the most severe cases, symptoms are evident in infancy, including facial paresis. In milder cases, significant clinical features may not become apparent until the second or third decade of life. The neurological findings and hearing loss are progressive. In the most severe cases, increased intracranial pressure and nerve compression can become life-threatening.

Treatment Prognosis: The progressive nature of the skeletal changes is intractable, but if not severe, the effects on the quality of life may be relatively mild, especially early in the expression of the disorder. Palliative treatment and surgical management are difficult because of the continuous production of new bone. Initial hearing loss will respond well to amplification, but the benefit may eventually be lost.

Differential Diagnosis: Progressive thickening of bone with craniofacial changes is common in the small number of syndromes categorized as osteochondrodysplasias, including **craniometaphyseal dysplasia, frontometaphyseal dysplasia,** and **craniodiaphyseal dysplasia.** Each has its own characteristic type of progression and effects on the long bones and cranium so that the diagnosis can be differentiated by radiographic study.

V

Velo-Cardio-Facial Syndrome (VCFS)

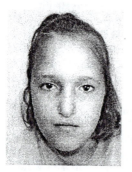 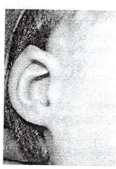 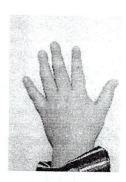

Velo-cardio-facial syndrome: Characteristic appearance of the face, showing a vertically long face, pear-shaped nose, overfolded helices on the ears with attached lobules (center), and small hands with tapered digits (right).

Also Known As: DiGeorge sequence (DGS), Cayler syndrome, conotruncal anomalies face syndrome, Sedlačková syndrome, 22q11 deletion syndrome, CATCH 22 (note: though this term has been applied by some clinicians, it has a pejorative connotation in its attempt at humor and should be avoided as a diagnostic label).

Velo-cardio-facial syndrome (VCFS) is probably the second most common multiple anomaly syndrome in humans with an estimated population prevalence of 1:2,000 people and a birth incidence which is undoubtedly higher, because some babies do not survive the neonatal period. VCFS has perhaps the most expansive phenotype of any multiple anomaly syndrome with over 180 clinical features already described. The syndrome was initially delineated because of the association of congenital heart disease, severe hypernasality, and learning disabilities. A small interstitial chromosomal deletion from the long arm of chromosome 22 at the q11.2 band was identified in 1992, at the same time psychiatric disorders became delineated as a common feature of the syndrome. Some type of communicative disorder is present in nearly all cases, including hypernasality, articulation impairment, language disorders, voice disorders, and conductive, sensorineural, or mixed hearing loss. It has been estimated that at least 5% of all patients in cleft palate clinics have this syndrome.

Major System(s) Affected:

Heart, vascular, craniofacial, central nervous system, skeletal, renal, immune, metabolic, limb, mental, cognitive, digestive, respiratory, genitourinary.

Etiology: A deletion of a small segment of the long arm of chromosome 22 at the 22q11.2 band. The deletion is typically approximately 3 million base pairs in length which encompasses many genes, but it is still not known if the syndrome is a contiguous gene or single gene deletion syndrome. The expression of the syndrome is inherited in an autosomal dominant manner with 100% penetrance. No imprinting or anticipation has been noted.

Quick Clues: A history of nasal vomiting is common. The presence of overfolded and adherent helices is a strong indication of the diagnosis of VCFS.

Hearing Disorders: Conductive, mixed, and sensorineural hearing loss have all been observed in VCFS. Conductive hearing loss is typically secondary to chronic middle ear effusion. Middle ear effusion is caused by both immune disorders and cleft palate. Sensorineural hearing loss occurs in at least 15% of cases and is most often unilateral and mild to moderate, but severe or profound bilateral loss has also been documented. An exaggerated startle response and phobic reaction to loud noises are common, but hyperacusis has not been found.

Speech Disorders: Severe articulation impairment, usually characterized by gross glottal stop substitutions when velopharyngeal insufficiency is present; velopharyngeal insufficiency (usually severe).

Feeding Disorders: There is often copious nasal regurgitation during feeding in the neonatal period, which may persist into early childhood. Though pH probes will register strongly positive, this finding should not be confused with reflux. Classic gastro-esophageal reflux does occur in some older children with VCFS, but the problem in infancy is significant emesis. Because of the combined effects of hypotonia and retrognathia, airway obstruction may also occur during feeding which will compromise efforts to nurse efficiently.

Voice Disorders: High pitched voice; hoarseness; breathiness.

Resonance Disorders: Hypernasality (usually severe).

Language Disorders: Language impairment (usually mild delay) with marked catch-up in language development between 3 and 4 years of age.

Other Clinical Features: Platybasia (flat skull base); asymmetric crying facies in infancy; structurally asymmetric face; functionally asymmetric face; vertical maxillary excess (long face); straight facial profile; congenitally missing teeth; small teeth; enamel hypoplasia (primary dentition); hypotonic flaccid facies; downturned oral commissures; cleft lip (uncommon); microcephaly; small posterior cranial fossa; tortuous retinal vessels; suborbital congestion ("allergic shiners"); strabismus; narrow palpebral fissures; posterior embryotoxon; small optic disk; prominent corneal nerves; cataract; iris nodules; iris coloboma (uncommon); retinal coloboma (uncommon); small eyes; mild orbital hypertelorism; mild orbital dystopia; puffy eyelids; overfolded helix; attached auricular lobules; protuberant cup-shaped ears; small ears; mildly asymmetric ears; ear tags or pits (uncommon); narrow external ear canals; prominent nasal bridge; bulbous nasal tip; mildly separated nasal domes (appearing bifid); pinched alar base; narrow nostrils; VSD (ventricular septal defect); ASD (atrial septal defect); pulmonic atresia or stenosis; tetralogy of Fallot; right-sided aorta; truncus arteriosus; PDA (patent ductus arteriosus); interrupted aorta; coarctation of the aorta; aortic valve anomalies; aberrant subclavian arteries; vascular ring; anomalous origin of carotid artery; transposition of the great vessels; tricuspid atresia; medially displaced internal carotid arteries; tortuous, kinked, absent, or accessory internal carotids; jugular vein anomalies; absence of vertebral artery (unilateral); low bifurcation of common carotid; tortuous or kinked vertebral arteries; Reynaud's phenomenon; small veins; circle of Willis anomalies; periventricular cysts (mostly at anterior horns); small cerebellar vermis; cerebellar hypoplasia/dysgenesis; white matter hyperintensities on MR examination; generalized hypotonia; seizures; strokes; spina bifida/meningomyelocele; mild developmental delay; enlarged Sylvian fissure; upper airway obstruction in infancy; absent or small adenoids; laryngeal web (anterior); large pharyngeal airway; laryngomalacia; arytenoid hyperplasia; pharyngeal hypotonia; asymmetric pharyngeal movement; thin pharyngeal muscle; unilateral vocal cord paresis; hypoplastic, aplastic, or cystic kidneys; Hirschsprung aganglionic megacolon has been reported in several cases; inguinal hernias; umbilical hernias; malrotation of the bowel; diaphragmatic hernia has been found in several cases; anal anomalies (displaced, imperforate); small hands and feet; tapered digits; short fingernails and toenails; rough, red, scaly skin on hands and feet; morphea; finger contractures; triphalangeal thumbs; polydactyly (both preaxial and postaxial); soft tissue syndactyly, especially of toes 2 and 3; feeding difficulty; failure-to-thrive; nasal vomiting; gastroesophageal reflux; nasal regurgitation; irritability; chronic constipation; learning disabilities (math concept, reading comprehension, problem-solving) with concrete thinking and difficulty with abstraction; occasional mild mental retardation; ADD or ADHD; thrombocytopenia; Bernard-Soulier disease; juvenile rheumatoid arthritis; mental illness, usually bipolar affective disorder; with rapid or ultrarapid cycling of mood disorder; schizoaffective disorder; impulsiveness; flat affect; dysthymia, cyclothymia; social immaturity; obsessive compulsive disorder; generalized anxiety disorder; phobias; frequent upper respiratory infections; frequent lower airway disease (pneumonia, bronchitis); reduced T cell populations; reduced thymic hormone; reactive airway disease or asthma; hypospadias; cryptorchidism; urethral reflux; hypocalcemia; hypoparathyroidism; pseudohypoparathyroidism; hypothyroidism; mild growth deficiency, relative small stature; absent or hypoplastic thymus; hypoplastic pituitary gland; scoliosis; hemivertebrae; spina bifida occulta; butterfly vertebrae; fused vertebrae (mostly cervical); tethered spinal cord; syrinx; osteopenia; Sprengel anomaly; talipes equinovarus (club foot); small skeletal muscles; joint dislocations; chronic leg pains; flat foot arches; hyperextensible and lax joints; extra ribs; rib fusion; abundant scalp hair; thin appearing skin (venous patterns easily visible); Robin sequence; DiGeorge sequence; Potter sequence; occasional **CHARGE association.**

Natural History: Early development of children with VCFS is marked by mild delay, with expressive language often showing a slightly larger lag than other milestones. Velopharyngeal insufficiency is common and usually leads to gross glottal stop subsitutions, which makes speech largely unintelligible. However, children with VCFS often show a dramatic spurt in development between 3 and 4 years of age. Early cognition is usually within normal limits, but learning disabilities involving abstraction and problem solving become evident in primary school and may be accompanied by a drop in IQ score, especially on Performance scales. School performance may be normal in early grades and deteriorate as the learning disorders become more obvious and subject matter becomes more difficult. Attention disorders may become evident in childhood, but often do not respond well to stimulants such as methylphenidate or dexedrine. Onset of psychiatric disorders often occurs in adolescence or young adult life, although in some cases, childhood psychiatric illness has been reported. Chronic respiratory and middle ear infections are most severe in early childhood (2 to 5 years of age) and gradually diminish in later childhood years.

Treatment Prognosis: A combination of speech therapy and surgical reconstruction of the velopharyngeal valve can result in normal speech in most cases. Learning problems respond best to repeated drill, which is also most effective during speech therapy. Psychiatric problems may progress in adult years to the point of psychosis.

Differential Diagnosis: There are many multiple syndromes with the combination of heart anomalies and cleft palate, including **Niikawa-Kuroki syndrome** (Kabuki make-up syndrome), **fetal alcohol syndrome,** and **CHARGE association.** There are also facial similarities between VCFS and **Langer-Giedion syndrome.** Mild orbital hypertelorism may occur in VCFS which, when in association with hypospadias and feeding difficulties, may lead clinicians to suspect **Opitz syndrome** (the G/BBB syndrome), which is an X-linked disorder. However, the large number of potential anomalies in VCFS can lead clinicians to search for additional phenotypic features prior to requesting FISH studies.

Waardenburg Syndrome

Also Known As: Waardenburg syndrome, type I.

Although primarily recognized as a syndrome of hearing loss, Waardenburg syndrome was originally delineated as a genetic disorder of the eyes. Until recently, Waardenburg syndrome was a single syndromic entity, but recently a number of separate disorders have been delineated representing distinct multiple anomalies with different etiologies. Waardenburg syndrome, type I is the disorder most commonly recognized as the "classic" phenotype and is the most common syndrome of its type (pigmentary and hearing disorders), associated with hearing loss. There are 5 different subtypes of "Waardenburg" syndromes, (type I, type IIA, type IIB, type III, and type IV). All have sensorineural hearing loss except type IV, also known as Waardenburg-Shah syndrome. It is estimated that 2 to 5% of people with congenital sensorineural hearing loss have a "Waardenburg" syndrome.

Major System(s) Affected: Integument; ocular; craniofacial; gastrointestinal; genitourinary; central nervous system.

Etiology: Autosomal dominant inheritance. The gene, *PAX3*, has been mapped to 2q35.

Quick Clues: Heterochromia iridium (two different colored eyes) and a white forelock are the obvious clues to the diagnosis of Waardenburg syndrome. However, the white forelock is not present throughout life in some cases, and is completely absent in others.

Hearing Disorders: Sensorineural hearing loss is present in approximately a quarter of patients with Waardenburg syndrome, type I. The hearing loss is variable, and may be either unilateral or bilateral. The majority of cases are bilateral. Severity also varies from mild to profound. The loss is not typically progressive. Affected frequencies also vary with some patients having residual low frequency hearing, others having upward sloping audiograms, and still others U-shaped. Vestibular abnormalities are present in some cases, but probably not the majority. The cochlea is typically hypoplastic in those cases with hearing loss, and anomalies or absence of the semicircular canals have been noted in some cases.

Speech Disorders: Articulation may be impaired in cases with cleft lip and palate. In others, severe or profound hearing loss may result in speech impairment.

Feeding Disorders: Feeding may be impaired in cases with cleft palate or with Hirschsprung megacolon.

Voice Disorders: Voice disorders have not been reported or observed in Waardenburg syndrome, type I.

Resonance Disorders: Hypernasality may be present in cases with cleft palate.

Language Disorders: Language may be affected by hearing loss.

Other Clinical Features:

> **Integument:** white forelock; white eyelashes; premature depigmentation of the scalp hair;

> **Ocular:** heterochromia iridium; telecanthus; depigmented fundus;

> **Craniofacial: cleft** lip and palate;

> **Gastrointestinal:** Hirschsprung aganglionic megacolon;

> **Genitourinary:** vaginal hypoplasia;

> **Central nervous system:** spina bifida; meningomyelocele;

> **Other:** rhabdomyosarcoma.

Natural History: The majority of the anomalies associated with Waardenburg syndrome, type I are congenital and static. When present, Hirschsprung aganglionic megacolon presents as severe constipation and slow clearance of the gut or impaction of the stool. There is premature graying of the hair that will mask the presence of the white forelock.

Treatment Prognosis: The anomalies associated with Waardenburg syndrome, type I are amenable to treatment, including surgical correction of the Hirschsprung aganglionic megacolon and amplification for hearing loss. Rhabdom-yosarcoma is treatable when detected early. The general prognosis is good.

Differential Diagnosis: Pigmentary anomalies are also present in the other subtypes of Waardenburg syndrome, as well as in a number of rare autosomal recessive disorders syndromes that have been isolated to a small number of individuals and families.

Waardenburg Syndrome, Type IIA

Also Known As: Waardenburg syndrome, type II.

Waardenburg syndrome, type IIA was initially differentiated from Waardenburg syndrome, type I because of the absence of telecanthus (dystopia canthorum). Hearing loss is far more common in type IIA than in type I.

Major System(s) Affected: Integument; ocular; craniofacial; gastrointestinal; genitourinary; central nervous system.

Etiology: Autosomal dominant inheritance. The gene has been mapped to 3p13.

Quick Clues: Heterochromia iridium (two different colored eyes) and a white forelock are the obvious clues to both Waardenburg type I and Waardenburg type IIA. The presence or absence of telecanthus is what largely differentiates the two sub types.

Hearing Disorders: Sensorineural hearing loss is present in ap-proximately half of patients with Waardenburg syndrome, type IIA. The hearing loss, as in type I, is variable in severity and is occasionally progressive. Vestibular abnormalities have been reported. The cochlea is typically hypoplastic in those cases with hearing loss, and anomalies of the semicircular canals have been noted.

Speech Disorders: Articulation may be impaired in cases with cleft lip and palate. In others, severe or profound hearing loss may result in speech impairment.

Feeding Disorders: Feeding may be impaired in cases with cleft palate or with Hirschsprung megacolon.

Voice Disorders: Voice disorders have not been reported or observed in Waardenburg syndrome, type IIA.

Resonance Disorders: Hypernasality may be present in cases with cleft palate.

Language Disorders: Language may be affected by hearing loss.

Other Clinical Features:

> **Integument:** white forelock; white eyelashes; premature depigmentation of the scalp hair;

> **Ocular:** heterochromia iridium; depigmented fundus;

> **Craniofacial:** cleft lip and palate; broad nasal root; short philtrum;

> **Gastrointestinal:** Hirschsprung aganglionic megacolon (uncommon);

> **Genitourinary:** vaginal hypoplasia;

> **Central nervous system:** spina bifida; meningomyelocele;

> **Other:** rhabdomyosarcoma.

Natural History: The majority of the anomalies associated with Waardenburg syndrome, type IIA are congenital and static. When present, Hirschsprung aganglionic megacolon presents as severe constipation and slow clearance of the gut or impaction of the stool. There is premature graying of the hair that will mask the presence of the white forelock. Hearing loss has been reported to be progressive in some cases.

Treatment Prognosis: The anomalies associated with Waardenburg syndrome, type IIA are amenable to treatment, including surgical correction of the Hirschsprung aganglionic megacolon and amplification for hearing loss. Rhabdomyosarcoma is treatable when detected early. The general prognosis is good.

Differential Diagnosis: Pigmentary anomalies are also present in the other subtypes of Waardenburg syndrome, as well as in a number of rare autosomal recessive disorders syndromes that have been isolated to a small number of individuals and families.

W

Waardenburg Syndrome with Ocular Albinism

Also Known As: Waardenburg syndrome, type II with ocular albinism.

Waardenburg syndrome with ocular albinism is a rare variant of this class of pigmentary disorders with hearing loss and is probably caused by more than a single mutation.

Major System(s) Affected: Integument; ocular.

Etiology: Autosomal dominant inheritance. Genes have been mapped to 11q and 3p.

Quick Clues: Translucent iris and nystagmus with multiple lentigines on the skin are clues to Waardenburg with ocular albinism.

Hearing Disorders: Sensorineural hearing loss and vestibular hypofunction are common.

Speech Disorders: Severe or profound hearing loss may result in speech impairment.

Feeding Disorders: Feeding is not impaired.

Voice Disorders: Voice disorders have not been reported or observed.

Resonance Disorders: Resonance disorders are not found unless caused by congenital deafness.

Language Disorders: Language may be affected by hearing loss.

Other Clinical Features:

> **Integument:** multiple lentigines; depigmentation of the skin;

> **Ocular:** translucent irises; albinism of the fundus; nystagmus; photophobia; visual impairment; strabismus; optic nerve dysplasia.

Natural History: The anomalies associated with Waardenburg syndrome with ocular albinism are congenital and static. Albinism and depigmentation may result in skin damage if exposed to the sun.

Treatment Prognosis: Amplification for hearing loss is recommended. Visual acuity is impaired and requires refraction.

Differential Diagnosis: Lentigines and sensorineural hearing loss are found in **multiple lentigines (LEOPARD) syndrome.** There are several genetic and syndromic forms of albinism, as well.

Wildervanck Syndrome

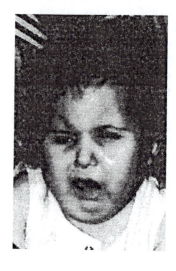

Wildervanck syndrome: Note facial asymmetry.

Also Known As: Cervico-oculo-acoustic syndrome.

Wildervanck syndrome is an underrecognized disorder that has facial asymmetry, spinal anomalies, hearing loss, and respiratory compromise as consistent clinical features. The disorder could be confused for **oculo-auriculo-vertebral dysplasia** because of the phenotypic overlap.

Major System(s) Affected: Craniofacial; ocular; musculoskeletal; neurologic; growth.

Etiology: Autosomal dominant inheritance. The gene has not been mapped or identified.

Quick Clues: The association of limited head movement and Duane syndrome should lead to the suspicion of Wildervanck syndrome.

Hearing Disorders: Hearing loss is common in Wildervanck syndrome and, because it is often unilateral, it may be underestimated in frequency. Purely sensorineural, purely conductive, and mixed hearing loss have all been documented. Anomalies that have been identified include ossicular malformations, stapes fixation, microtia, and Mondini anomaly. Vestibular dysfunction has also been noted.

Speech Disorders: Speech disorders are highly variable, ranging from severe delay and impairment to essentially normal speech. Speech is affected by sensorineural hearing loss, malocclusion, airway compromise, and cognitive impairment, none of which are constant findings in the syndrome, nor are they mutually exclusive. Normal intellect is the norm in the syndrome, but cognitive impairment has been observed. Posterior airway obstruction can cause fronting and tongue protrusion during speech. Malocclusion secondary to facial asymmetry and occasional anterior skeletal open-bite (growth changes caused by airway obstruction) result in obligatory placement errors and distortions.

Feeding Disorders: Infant and early childhood feeding can be severely compromised by airway obstruction caused by a small pharyngeal airway and retrognathia with a short neck that reduces the vertical dimensions of the airway. Failure-to-thrive may result from airway obstruction, but will resolve with management of the airway disorder. Limited oral opening in some cases may further exacerbate the problem.

Voice Disorders: Voice may be hoarse secondary to chronic airway obstruction causing the lymphoid tissue, even when normal in size, to crowd the pharynx and increase the amount of congestion.

Resonance Disorders: Both hyponasality and hypernasality have been observed. Hyponasality is secondary to obstruction of an already small airway by the adenoids and/or tonsils. Hypernasality has been observed by the author in a single case that had a submucous cleft palate. Oral resonance is also severely impaired by the combination of a small pharyngeal airway and a vertically short airway. Oral resonance is often muffled.

Language Disorders: Language development is usually normal, but in cases with cognitive impairment, language will be delayed.

Other Clinical Features:

Craniofacial: craniofacial asymmetry; variable external ear anomalies; maxillary and mandibular hypoplasia; acute

W

angulation of the cranial base; low-set, posteriorly rotated ears; low posterior hairline; cleft palate or submucous cleft palate;

Ocular: unilateral or bilateral Duane syndrome (abducens palsy);

Musculoskeletal: cervical spine malformations, including Klippel-Feil anomaly, vertebral fusions, and spina bifida occulta; Sprengel shoulder; torticollis;

Neurologic: occasional cognitive impairment;

Growth: occasional short stature.

Natural History: All anomalies are present at birth, including the hearing loss, and are nonprogressive.

Treatment Prognosis: With proper management of the hearing loss and airway obstruction, the prognosis is generally good. Eventual craniofacial reconstruction can eliminate the malocclusion, but must be deferred until teen years. However, mandibular distraction is probably applicable to the disorder and may also have a positive effect on airway obstruction.

Differential Diagnosis: Oculo-auriculo-vertebral dysplasia has many of the same phenotypic features as Wildervanck syndrome, including spinal anomalies, external ear anomalies, hearing loss (usually conductive), and facial asymmetry. Sensorineural hearing loss with external ear anomalies is found in **BOR syndrome.** However, the Klippel-Feil anomaly and Duane palsy will differentiate Wildervanck syndrome.

Williams Syndrome

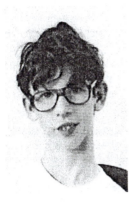

Williams syndrome: Facial appearance of an adolescent with Williams syndrome.

Also Known As: Williams-Beuren syndrome, elfin facies with hypercalcemia.

Williams syndrome is one of the more easily recognizable syndromes with a birth frequency of approximately 1:10,000 to 1:15,000. Williams syndrome has particular interest for speech-language pathologists because of its unique language phenotype. Children with Williams syndrome, essentially all of whom are mentally retarded, have very sophisticated language structure.

Major system(s) affected: Central nervous system; craniofa-cial; dental; cardiac; growth; musculoskeletal; genitourinary; gastrointestinal; endocrine.

Etiology: Interstitial deletion from the long arm of chromosome 7 at 7q11.2, encompassing the elastin gene, labeled as *ELN*.

Quick Clues: A wide mouth and thick lips are a nearly constant finding in Williams syndrome.

Hearing Disorders: Hyperacusis has been reported as a common finding in Williams syndrome, but it is unclear if this phenomenon is one of a significant startle response versus true sound sensitivity.

309

W

Hearing loss is not a primary feature of Williams syndrome, although chronic middle ear effusion has been reported with associated temporary conductive hearing loss.

Speech Disorders: Articulation may be slightly slurred, and speech rate is often rapid, sometimes causing mild unintelligibility. However, in many cases, articulation skills are quite good with normal intelligibility.

Feeding Disorders: Early failure-to-thrive is common in Williams syndrome and is often attributed to hypotonia and heart anomalies.

Voice Disorders: Voice is often harsh and hoarse.

Resonance Disorders: Resonance is normal.

Language Disorders: Developmental delay is nearly always present with many affected individuals being mildly or moderately retarded, others having borderline normal intellect. When language develops, there is an abundant use of echolalia and cliches. The structure of language use is sophisticated, but the content of the message is often difficult to extract and sometimes makes little sense. Syntax is often impaired. Manner and affect are best described as affable and very interactive, but are accompanied by hyperactivity and impulsivity with poor behavioral control.

Other Clinical Features:

Central nervous system: hypotonia, cognitive impairment, strokes, seizures, ADD and ADHD;

Craniofacial: thick lips; long philtrum; anteverted nostrils; epicanthal folds; puffy periorbital area; flaring of the eyebrows; wide mouth;

Dental: hypodontia; microdontia;

Cardiac: supravalvular aortic stenosis; mitral valve prolapse; atrial septal defect; ventriculoseptal defect; pulmonary stenosis;

Growth: short stature;

Musculoskeletal: rib anomalies; limitation of joints; scoliosis; inguinal hernia;

Genitourinary: urinary tract infections; kidney anomalies; urethral stenosis;

Gastrointestinal: chronic constipation; diverticulosis;

Endocrine: hypercalcemia.

Natural History: Developmental milestones are universally delayed, and many infants with Williams syndrome are irritable. In childhood, they become overly friendly and often crave the attention of adults and other children. Although the large majority are cognitively impaired, their sophisticated language structure often makes their performance seem better than it truly is. Many children and adults with Williams syndrome have a strong affinity for music and some have been labeled as "savants" because they often have strong memories for music, names, and facts. Life expectancy is not impaired unless heart anomalies or other vascular structural defects are severe.

Treatment Prognosis: Children with Williams syndrome can learn and they do not have the same "plateau" effect as is seen in Down syndrome. Many of the more severely retarded individuals may require a sheltered or semi-sheltered environment, but others with higher cognitive function can be relatively independent.

Differential Diagnosis: The phenotype of Williams syndrome is distinct and is not easily confused with other disorders.

W

Index

CPSIA information can be obtained
at www.ICGtesting.com
Printed in the USA
FFOW04n1150140114
3099FF